AF882120

Easy Vegan Sauces

Simple Plant-Based Sauce Recipes for Everyday Living

Easy Vegan Sauces

Simple Plant-Based Sauce Recipes for Everyday Living

Copyright © 2026 by Kate Witkowski

Witkowski Publishing

ISBN: 978-1-950114-24-5

All rights reserved.

No part of this workbook may be reproduced, distributed, or transmitted in any form or by any means, including photocopying, recording, or other electronic or mechanical methods, without prior written permission from the publisher, except in the case of brief quotations embodied in critical reviews and certain other noncommercial uses permitted by copyright law.

This book is intended for personal use only.

Printed in the United States of America.

Contact:
Kate Witkowski

Kate Witkowski

www.cleaneatsstreet.com

Kate@KateWitkowski.com

Clean Eats Street

A Note Before You Begin

This book was created to solve one very practical problem:

How do you make everyday meals taste good—consistently—without starting from scratch every time?

Sauces are the quiet backbone of cooking. They turn simple ingredients into complete meals, help you repeat dishes without boredom, and make plant-based cooking feel satisfying rather than complicated.

Easy Vegan Sauces is designed as a working reference you can return to again and again. You don't need to cook through it in order, memorize anything, or follow it cover to cover. Use it the way real kitchens work—open to the section you need, make what fits your meal, and move on.

How This Book Is Designed to Be Used

This is not a traditional cookbook built around menus or finished plates. It's a **building-block system**.

Inside, you'll find sauces organized by type—tomato-based, creamy blends, curries, gravies, marinades, dressings, drizzles, and more—so you can quickly match a sauce to what you're already cooking.

Each recipe is written to be:

- Flexible
- Adaptable
- Easy to scale up or down
- Suitable for everyday meals, not special occasions

You can follow the recipes exactly or treat them as starting points. Both approaches are encouraged.

What You'll Find Inside

This book includes more than 100 plant-based sauces, spreads, dressings, and flavor bases designed to work across a wide range of meals.

You'll find:

- Everyday tomato sauces that work for pasta, grains, and vegetables
- Creamy dairy-free sauces made from cashews, beans, tofu, and seeds
- Bold curry sauces and global flavor blends
- Comfort-style gravies and savory sauces
- Marinades, vinaigrettes, and drizzles for quick flavor boosts
- Condiments, glazes, and finishing sauces
- Foundational techniques for building and balancing flavor

Later sections explain how ingredients like nuts, seeds, herbs, spices, and nutritional yeast work together—so you can confidently adjust, customize, and create your own sauces over time.

A Simple Philosophy

The recipes in this book are intentionally generous. Many make enough sauce to coat a full 16-ounce box of pasta or serve multiple meals. This allows you to cook once and use the sauce in different ways throughout the week.

Nothing here is meant to be rigid.

Use what you have.
Adjust to taste.
Swap ingredients when needed.
Repeat what works for you.

The goal is not perfection—it's familiarity.

One Last Thought

When meals feel repetitive or uninspired, it's often not the main ingredient that needs changing—it's the flavor behind it.

Sauces give you range without complexity. They help you cook with confidence, even on busy days, using ingredients you already know.

This book is meant to live in your kitchen, not on a shelf.

Open it often. Skip around. Make it yours.

TABLE OF CONTENTS

A Note Before You Begin 3

How This Book Is Designed to Be Used 3

What You'll Find Inside 4

A Simple Philosophy 4

One Last Thought 5

Notes About the Recipes 16

1. How to Create Your Own Sauce 19

Flavor Patterns 22

Nutritional Yeast and Soaked Nuts- The Inside Scoop 23

2. Tomato Based Sauces 27

Classic Marinara Sauce 28

Roasted Red Pepper Sauce I 30

Roasted Red Pepper Sauce II 32

Creamy Garlic Tomato Sauce 33

Smoky Tomato Paprika Sauce 34

Creamy Smoky Arrabbiata 35

Mediterranean Olive and Capers Sauce 37

Tomato White Bean Cream Sauce 38

Fire Roasted Tomato Basil Sauce 39

3. Creamy Sauces and Cashew Blends 41

Classic Cashew Cream Sauce 42

Mushroom Cashew Cream Sauce 43

Garlic Tahini Cashew Cream Sauce 44

Coconut Curry Cashew Sauce 45

Lemon Dill Cashew Sauce 46

Creamy Dill Pasta Sauce 47

White Bean Alfredo Sauce 49
Creamy Cold Noodle Sauce 50
Lemon Pasta Salad Sauce 51
Miso Lemon Pasta Sauce 52
Cashew Cauliflower Alfredo 53
Lemon Caper Pasta Sauce 55
Walnut Mushroom Bolognese 56
Lemon Herb Orzo Sauce 57
Vegetable "Cream Sauce" Base 58
Creamy Spinach Pasta Sauce 59
Caramelized Onion Pasta Sauce 60
Sweet Corn Pasta Sauce 61
Green Goddess Pasta Sauce 62
Butternut or Pumpkin Cream Sauce 63
Creamy Artichoke Pasta Sauce 65
Lemon Parsley 'Butter' Sauce 66
Garlic White Bean 'Scampi' Sauce 67
Cashew Pesto Cream Sauce 68
Roasted Garlic Alfredo 69
Creamy Sunflower Seed Pasta Sauce 71
Lemon Tahini Pasta Sauce 72
Mushroom 'Marsala' Pasta Sauce 73
Caramelized Fennel Pasta Sauce 75
Zesty Roasted Lemon Sauce 76
Cashew 'Ricotta' Pasta Sauce 77
Creamy Garlic Herb Mushroom Sauce 78
Bruschetta Pasta Sauce 80

4. Curry Sauces 81

Thai Red Curry Coconut Sauce 82
Golden Curry Cashew Sauce 83
Tomato Coconut Curry Sauce 84
Green Herb Coconut Curry Sauce 85
Sweet Potato Curry Sauce 86

5. Tofu-Based and Protein-Boosted Sauces 87
Silken Tofu Alfredo 88
Tofu Garlic Lemon Sauce 89
Spicy Tofu Aioli 90
Creamy Basil Tofu Sauce 91
Smoky Tofu Cream 92

6. Nut and Seed-Based Sauces 93
Peanut Satay Sauce 94
Almond Ginger Sauce 95
Sunflower Seed Dressing 96
Sesame Miso Sauce 97
Walnut and Roasted Garlic Spread 98

7. Comfort Sauces and Gravies 99
Homemade Cranberry Sauce 100
Slow Cooker Cranberry Sauce 101
Savory Cranberry Herb Gravy 102
Salisbury Style Slow Cooker Gravy 103
Slow Cooker Savory Mushroom Gravy 104
Cashew Cream Comfort Gravy 106
Tofu Cream Country Gravy 107
Mediterranean Herb Gravy 108
Caramelized Onion Gravy 109

Peppercorn Gravy 110
Miso Rosemary Gravy 111
Smoky Paprika Gravy 112
Garlic Sage Gravy 113
Herb Tahini Gravy 114
Creamy Garlic Gravy 115
Onion Miso Gravy 116
Coconut Pepper Gravy 117
Rosemary Shallot Gravy 118
5. Homemade "Packet-Style" Mixes 119
Ranch Seasoning Mix 120
Dried Onion Soup Mix 121
Brown Gravy Mix 122
Simple Dry Rub for Vegetables and Tofu 123
Preserved Lemon Herb Blend 124
Dill Herb Seasoning Mix 125
9. Condiment Sauces and Glazes 126
Simple Mustard Sauce 127
Sweet Chili Sauce 128
Classic BBQ Sauce 129
Peach BBQ Sauce 130
Mango BBQ Sauce 131
Smoky Maple BBQ Sauce 132
Sweet and Smoky BBQ Sauce 133
Korean-Style Gochujang BBQ Sauce 134
Classic Vegan Mayo (Base Recipe) 135
Chipotle Mayo 136

Chili Lime Mayo....137
Garlic Herb Mayo....138
Garlic Aioli Mayo....139
Dijon Mayo....140
Horseradish Mayo....141
10. Mediterranean Sauces....142
Sidebar: About Mediterranean Sauces....143
Romesco Sauce....144
Mediterranean Olive and Herb Sauce....145
Mediterranean Tomato Caper Sauce....146
Lemon Tahini Mediterranean Drizzle....147
Tomato Caper Garlic Sauce....148
Herbed Yogurt Tahini Mediterranean Blend....149
Muhammara (Roasted Pepper and Walnut Sauce)....150
Lemon Garlic Gremolata....151
Tzatziki Style Cucumber Yogurt....152
Lemon Oregano Mediterranean Marinade....153
Basil Walnut Pesto....154
11. Everyday Sauces and Glazes....155
Peanut Lime Sauce....156
Miso Tahini Sauce....157
Ginger Scallion Sauce....158
Dill Garlic Sauce....159
Creamy Dill Sauce....161
Creamy Dill Sauce with Chopped Pickles....162
Teriyaki Sauce....163
Pineapple Ginger Teriyaki Sauce....164

Teriyaki Glaze 165
Maple Mustard Glaze 166
Brown Sugar Glaze 167
Maple Chipotle Glaze 168
12. Marinades 169
Soy Ginger Marinade 170
Sweet Garlic Marinade 171
Sesame Orange Marinade 172
Chili Lime Marinade 173
Lemon Mustard Herb Marinade 174
Lemon Dill Marinade 175
13. Vinaigrettes 176
Classic Lemon Vinaigrette 177
Apple Cider Maple Dressing 178
Balsamic Dijon Vinaigrette 179
Orange Tahini Vinaigrette 180
Mediterranean Herb Vinaigrette 181
14. Creamy Dressings 182
Cashew Ranch Dressing 183
Tofu Caesar Dressing 184
Avocado Lime Dressing 185
Greek Yogurt Dill Dressing 186
Chipotle Cream Dressing 187
Carrot Ginger Dressing 188
Herb Tahini Dressing 189
15. Dips and Spreads 190
Classic Hummus (Base) 191

Roasted Red Pepper Hummus ... 192
Smoky Black Bean Dip ... 193
Creamy Spinach and Artichoke Dip ... 194
Edamame Ginger Spread ... 195
Creamy Dill Dip ... 196
16. Non-Dairy Yogurts and Cheeses ... 198
Coconut Yogurt (Base) ... 199
Almond Yogurt ... 200
Cashew Yogurt ... 201
Simple Tofu 'Ricotta' ... 202
Cashew 'Parmesan' ... 203
17. Flavor-Enhancing Add-Ons ... 204
Cashew 'La Crema' Sauce ... 205
Coconut Lime Drizzle ... 206
Balsamic Reduction ... 207
Maple Miso Butter ... 208
Garlic Confit ... 209
Lemon Herb Oil ... 210
Simple Parsley Herb Sauce ... 211
18. Drizzles ... 212
Chili Lime Oil ... 213
Tahini Drizzle ... 214
Balsamic Swirl ... 215
Sweet and Spicy Maple Glaze ... 216
19. Comfort Sauces ... 217
Potato Based 'Cheese' Sauce ... 218
Silky Tofu Based 'Cheese' Sauce ... 219

Cashew Blender 'Cheese' Sauce 220
White Bean 'Cheese' Sauce 221
How to Cook Beans from Scratch 222
Black Bean Sauce 225
Spicy Chipotle–Roasted Garlic Black Bean Sauce 227
Cilantro Lime Green Black Bean Sauce 228
Cashew Black Bean Queso 229
20. Fresh Classics 231
Classic Guacamole 232
Mild Fresh Salsa 233
Spicy Salsa Roja 234
Green Tomatillo Salsa (Salsa Verde) 235
Mock Sour 'Cream' 238
Chimichurri Sauce 239
Lemon Dill Tahini Sauce 240
Greek Style Dill Sauce (Vegan Tzatziki) 241
Dill Avocado Green Sauce 242
21. Jams and Marmalades 243
Classic Orange Marmalade 244
Strawberry Basil Jam 245
Mixed Berry Chia Jam 246
Sweet Pepper Jam 247
Peach Ginger Jam 248
Green Cilantro Chutney 249
Cranberry Apple Chutney 250
22. Dessert Drizzles 251
Hazelnut Chocolate Spread 252

Salted Caramel Date Sauce 253
Maple Ginger Sauce 254
Berry Balsamic Drizzle 255
Chocolate Sauce 256
Salted Chocolate Sauce 258
Orange Infused Chocolate Sauce 259
Mint Chocolate Sauce 260
Mocha Chocolate Sauce 261
Spiced Mexican Chocolate Sauce 262
Maple Cinnamon Chocolate Sauce 263
Coconut Almond Chocolate Sauce 264
23. Herbs 265
Fresh vs. Dried: When and Why 265
Infusing Oils and Dressings with Herbs 266
Growing and Storing Fresh Herbs 266
Herb Pairing Guide 267
24. Spices 268
The Role of Spices in Vegan Cooking 268
Italian Herb Blend 270
Curry Spice Blend 271
Smoky BBQ Rub 272
Sweet Spice Mix 273
25. Nuts and Seeds 274
How to Toast, Grind and Store 274
Homemade Nut or Seed Butter 276
Quick Nut Milk (No Soak Version) 277
Savory Nut and Seed Sprinkle 278

Sweet Spice Nut Crumble 279
26. Infused Waters 280
Cucumber-Mint-Lime Water 281
Strawberry-Basil Water 281
Citrus-Ginger Water 281
Pineapple-Mint Water 282
Blueberry-Lavender Water 282
27. Bringing It All Together 283
How to Combine Sauces, Dressings and Add-Ons 283
Quick Flavor Maps 284
Sample "Staples Week" 284
The "Make It Yours Ideas" Customization Guide 285
Conversion and Measurement Reference 285
Closing Notes 286

Notes About the Recipes

1. Recipe Yields and Large Quantities

Some of the recipes — especially tomato-based sauces and creamy sauces — use large quantities of tomatoes, vegetables, or cashews. This is intentional. I designed these recipes to make a generous amount of sauce that fully coats a 16-ounce box of pasta. If you prefer lighter coverage or want a smaller batch, simply cut the recipe in half. The flavor and consistency will remain the same.

2. Vegan Ingredients are a Personal Choice

These recipes are only as vegan as the ingredients you choose.

For example:

- Using broccoli packaged in a butter sauce is not vegan.
- Using honey instead of maple syrup is not vegan.
- Serving bread made with eggs or dairy will not keep the meal fully vegan.

The bottom line: you choose what works best for your kitchen and lifestyle.

3. Adjusting Thickness & Consistency

Every sauce can be thickened or thinned based on your preference.

- To thin a sauce: add water, broth, plant milk or reserved pasta water 1–2 tablespoons at a time.
- To thicken a sauce: simmer uncovered to reduce, or add extra cashews, beans, tahini, tomato paste or blended vegetables.
- To make sauces exceptionally smooth: blend in a high-speed blender or blend 30–60 seconds longer than you think you need.

4. **Sauce Flavor Balancing Tips**

Small adjustments can dramatically improve a sauce:

- Add acid (lemon, vinegar) to brighten and lift heavy flavors.
- Add sweetness (maple syrup, coconut sugar) to reduce bitterness or tame acidity.
- Add fat (olive oil, tahini, coconut milk) for richness and cohesion.
- Add umami (nutritional yeast, miso, tomato paste) for depth and savory roundness.

Taste as you go and adjust in small increments.

5. **Salt Levels Will Vary**

Salt requirements differ depending on:

- the brand of broth you use,
- whether your nuts or seeds are salted,
- added condiments (miso, soy sauce, capers, olives),
- your personal taste.

Salt conservatively at first and increase gradually.

6. **Use Water Content of Vegetables to Your Advantage**

Vegetables like tomatoes, zucchini, mushrooms, and onions release moisture as they cook. If your sauce becomes thinner than expected, simply:

- simmer uncovered to reduce, or
- add a small handful of cashews or a spoonful of tomato paste to bring it back into balance.

7. Storage & Freezing

Most sauces — especially tomato-based, cashew-based, and bean-based blends — freeze beautifully.

General guidelines:

- Refrigerate 4–5 days in an airtight container.
- Freeze 2–3 months.
- Thaw overnight in the refrigerator or warm on low heat while stirring.
- Add a splash of plant milk or broth after reheating to restore creaminess.

8. Ingredient Flexibility

Every sauce is adaptable:

- Swap cashews for sunflower seeds if nut-free.
- Replace coconut milk with plant milk to reduce richness.
- Use canned tomatoes when fresh tomatoes are not available.
- Use dried herbs if fresh herbs aren't on hand (1 teaspoon dried = ~1 tablespoon fresh).

Your kitchen, your rules.

9. Taste Before Serving

Because so many sauces involve blending, roasting, or reduction, the flavor intensifies as they cook. Always take a final taste and adjust:

- more lemon/vinegar,
- a touch of sweetness,
- a sprinkle of salt,
- an extra pinch of spice.

1. How to Create Your Own Sauce

A plantsy guide to building flavor with confidence

My mother always said, "*A recipe is only a suggestion, Kate — create food you love... unless your friend is coming for dinner.*" She also reminded me, "*If you know how to read, you know how to cook.*" Those two ideas became the foundation of everything I create for Plantsy Vegan Eats: recipes that work, with room for personalization, exploration, and creativity.

This book includes more than 100 sauces, drizzles, dressings, gravies, and flavor foundations. But a list of ingredients only turns into fabulous food when you start mixing and matching, trying new combinations, and adapting the recipes to your preferences. With a few guiding principles, the possibilities become endless.

Below is a flexible way to think about creating your own sauces. These are not rules — just starting points to spark your imagination in the kitchen.

Step 1: Choose Your Base

Most vegan sauces begin with one of three base categories. Each creates a different texture and flavor profile.

- *Cashew-Based* - Soak raw cashews. Blend with water, broth, or plant milk.
    - Creates thick, creamy sauces
    - Neutral flavor (easy to adapt)
    - Excellent for Alfredo-style sauces, cheese-style sauces, and dessert drizzles
- *Tofu-Based* - Blend soft or firm tofu with aromatics or seasonings.
    - Lighter than cashews but still creamy
    - High-protein base

- Ideal for aiolis, lighter cream sauces, herbed blends, dips, and yogurt-style sauces

- *Non-Dairy–Based* - Use vegan yogurt, sour cream, cream cheese, or coconut milk.
  - Quickest, most convenient base
  - Smooth and consistent textures
  - Perfect for sweet sauces, herb sauces, Mediterranean blends, and curry-inspired sauces

Step 2: Decide Your Direction — Sweet or Savory

Before adding anything else, ask yourself one simple question: *What direction should the sauce lean?*

- *Savory* - Think garlic, onion, herbs, spices, tomato paste, miso, vinegar, lemon juice, tahini, or broth.
- *Sweet* - Think maple syrup, coconut sugar, vanilla, fruit, citrus, cinnamon, or cocoa.

This single choice shapes the entire personality of your sauce.

Step 3: Consider the Purpose

Ask yourself what the sauce is for, and the decisions become easy.

- *What will it go on?*

Vegetables? Pasta? Grain bowls? Roasted potatoes? Beans? Tofu?

- *What consistency should it be?*

Smooth? Chunky? Thin? Thick? Spreadable? Drizzle-style?

- *Should the flavor be bold or subtle?*

Punchy and bright? Rich and creamy? Light and balanced?

- *Adjust texture intentionally:*
    - Add liquid to thin
    - Add nuts, seeds, tofu, or more base to thicken
    - Simmer to reduce
    - Add acid or herbs for brightness
    - Add sweetness to soften sharp edges

Texture matters just as much as flavor.

Step 4: Add Your Flavor Builders

Once you have your base, direction, and purpose, bring the sauce to life with these essentials:

- *Nutritional Yeast*
    - Adds umami and cheese-like depth.
    - Balances acidity and prevents savory sauces from tasting flat.
- *Plant Milk or Broth*
    - Adjusts texture while softening sharper flavors.
- *Herbs and Spices*
    - Fresh herbs = brightness and freshness
    - Dried herbs = warmth and depth
    - Spices = character (smoky, spicy, earthy, sweet, aromatic)
- *Acidic Ingredients*
    - Lemon juice, vinegar, tomato paste — all brighten and balance.
- *Fat Elements*
    - Olive oil, tahini, coconut milk, or vegan butter add body and richness.

Flavor Patterns

Peanut Sauce Base

Peanut butter + soy sauce + garlic + maple + lime

Perfect for:

- Noodle dishes
- Bowls
- Dips
- Glazes

Add-ons: chili paste, coconut milk, ginger, rice vinegar.

Gravy Base

Start with:

- Onion
- Garlic
- Broth
- Fat + flour roux

Flavor comes from:

- Ranch seasoning
- Onion soup mix
- Brown gravy mix

Dessert Sauce Base

Begin with a creamy base. Gently warm with combinations of:

- Fruit purées
- Plant milk
- Maple syrup or coconut sugar
- Cocoa
- Vanilla
- Cinnamon or nutmeg

Creates:

- Drizzles
- Glazes
- Pour-over sauces
- Chocolate or caramel-style blends

Nutritional Yeast and Soaked Nuts- The Inside Scoop

Nutritional Yeast and Soaked Nuts Are a Vegan Sauce Lover's Best Friend. Why? Vegan sauces rely on two quiet powerhouses that deliver richness, depth, and creaminess without dairy: nutritional yeast and soaked nuts. These two ingredients work together (or separately) to create the velvety textures and savory flavors that define many plant-based sauces. Understanding why they're so effective helps you confidently adapt recipes, troubleshoot textures, and create your own blends with ease.

Nutritional Yeast - The Flavor Builder

Nutritional yeast—often called "nooch"—is a deactivated yeast grown on molasses, harvested, and dried into flakes or powder. It's naturally rich in B-vitamins, protein, trace minerals, and glutamic acid, which is responsible for its unmistakable savory, "cheesy," umami quality.

What nutritional yeast does in sauces:

- Adds depth: A spoonful transforms a mild sauce into something rounder, fuller, and more satisfying.
- Boosts savoriness: It brings a gentle "cheese-like" flavor—never overpowering unless used in large amounts.
- Enhances creaminess: Even though it's dry, it thickens sauces slightly and gives your base a creamy, cohesive mouthfeel.
- Improves stability: In blended sauces, it helps emulsify fats and liquids, reducing separation.

You can use flakes or powder interchangeably; flakes blend smoothly once heated or puréed.

Soaked Nuts - The Cream Maker

Cashews, almonds, macadamias, pistachios, and even sunflower seeds can be transformed into luscious, dairy-free cream with one simple step: soaking. Nuts are naturally high in healthy fats, mild in flavor, and full of plant protein—an ideal combination for building body and silkiness in sauces.

Why Soaking Matters

- Softens the nut: Hydrated nuts blend more fully, creating a smoother, richer purée.
- Improves texture: A well-soaked cashew produces a velvety cream with no graininess.

- Reduces blending time: Soaking makes the process easier on your blender and reduces the need for constant scraping.
- Enhances digestibility: Hydration helps break down some naturally occurring compounds that can make nuts harder to digest.

How to Soak Nuts

You can soak most nuts in two easy ways:

1. Standard Soak (Best Texture):

   Cover the nuts with room-temperature water for 4–8 hours or overnight. Drain and rinse before blending.

2. Quick Soak (Fast Option):

   Pour hot water over the nuts and soak for 15–30 minutes. This shortcut works especially well for cashews.

Avoid soaking pistachios or walnuts for long periods—15–30 minutes is enough, or they may become bitter.

How to Blend for a Perfect Cream

To achieve the silkiest result:

1. Add the soaked nuts to the blender.
2. Add liquid slowly—vegetable broth, plant milk, or water.
3. Start on low, then move to high speed.
4. Blend until glossy, thick, and completely smooth.
5. Add more liquid to thin to your desired consistency.

A high-speed blender gives the best texture, but soaked nuts can become creamy even in a standard blender with extra blending time.

Why These Two Ingredients Work So Well Together

When nutritional yeast and soaked nuts appear in the same recipe, they create a powerful synergy:

- Nuts provide body and creaminess.
- Nutritional yeast brings the savory flavor notes that mimic cheese or deepen the base.
- Together they create sauces that feel indulgent but remain simple, wholesome, and dairy-free.

You can adjust each component depending on whether you want a sauce that's thick and rich (increase the nuts), more flavorful (add a bit more nutritional yeast), or lighter (thin the mixture with broth or water).

Try These Pairings and Ideas

- Add nutritional yeast to cashew cream for a quick cream sauce.
- Blend soaked almonds with lemon juice and nutritional yeast for a bright, tangy drizzle.
- Mix soaked cashews, garlic, vegetable broth, and yeast for a blender-style Alfredo.
- Stir nutritional yeast into any broth-based gravy for added depth.

Final Thoughts: Creativity Is the Secret Ingredient

Use the recipes in this book as inspiration — not limitation. Taste as you go. Adjust seasoning. Try new herbs and spices. Blend nuts and seeds for richness. Layer flavors from different sections. Mix Mediterranean with Thai, sweet with savory, creamy with spicy.

A recipe is a suggestion — and now you have the tools to create sauces that feel like *you*.

2. Tomato Based Sauces

Simple staples that turn grains, veggies, and plant proteins into craveable meals.

Bright, bold, and endlessly adaptable — these tomato sauces are the heart of so many vegan meals. Roasted fresh tomatoes, garlic, and herbs form the foundation for everything from simple marinara to complex smoky blends. They're perfect for tossing with pasta, layering over grains, or spooning onto roasted vegetables.

- Classic Marinara Sauce
- Roasted Red Pepper Sauce I
- Roasted Red Pepper Sauce II
- Creamy Garlic Tomato Sauce
- Smoky Tomato Paprika Sauce
- Creamy Smoky Arrabbiata Sauce
- Mediterranean Olive and Capers Sauce
- Tomato White Bean Cream Sauce
- Fire Roasted Tomato Basil Sauce

Classic Marinara Sauce

A timeless, slow-simmered marinara that blends roasted tomatoes, garlic, herbs, balsamic vinegar, and chili flakes into a rich, bright, deeply flavorful sauce. Perfect for pasta, grain bowls, roasted vegetables and layered bakes.

Makes About 4 cups | Prep Time 10 minutes | Cook Time 35 minutes

Ingredients

4 pounds ripe Roma or plum tomatoes, halved

12 garlic cloves, unpeeled

4 small yellow onions, peeled and quartered

8 tablespoons olive oil

4 teaspoons dried oregano

2 teaspoons dried basil or 4 tablespoons chopped fresh basil

2 teaspoons fine sea salt

1 teaspoon black pepper

2 teaspoons red pepper flakes

4 tablespoons tomato paste

4 tablespoons balsamic vinegar

4 teaspoons maple syrup

Directions

1. Preheat the oven to 400 degrees. Line a baking sheet with parchment paper.
2. Arrange the halved tomatoes cut side up and add the garlic cloves and quartered onions.
3. Drizzle with the olive oil and sprinkle with oregano, basil, salt, black pepper, and red pepper flakes.

4. Roast for 25 to 30 minutes, until the tomatoes collapse and the edges caramelize.
5. Transfer the roasted tomatoes, onions, and peeled garlic cloves to a saucepan.
6. Add the tomato paste, balsamic vinegar, and maple syrup.
7. Use an immersion blender to blend to your preferred texture — smooth or slightly chunky.
8. Warm over medium heat for 5 to 10 minutes to thicken and deepen the flavor.
9. Adjust salt, pepper, or balsamic as needed.

Pairs With

Spaghetti, rigatoni, lasagna layers, roasted eggplant, zucchini noodles, baked tofu, polenta bowls, or Italian-style casseroles.

Roasted Red Pepper Sauce I

Sweet, smoky, and silky-smooth — this roasted red pepper sauce blends fire-roasted peppers, garlic, smoked paprika, and a touch of nutritional yeast into a bright, versatile sauce perfect for pasta, wraps, bowls, and roasted vegetables.

Makes About 4 cups | Prep Time 10 minutes | Cook Time 20 minutes

Ingredients

12 large red bell peppers, halved and seeded

12 garlic cloves, unpeeled

8 tablespoons olive oil, divided

2 teaspoons smoked paprika

2 teaspoons fine sea salt

1 teaspoon black pepper

4 tablespoons tomato paste

2 cups unsweetened plant milk

4 tablespoons nutritional yeast

4 tablespoons lemon juice

2 teaspoons cayenne pepper

Directions

1. Preheat the oven to 425 degrees. Line a baking sheet with parchment paper.
2. Place the peppers cut side down on the sheet along with the garlic cloves.
3. Brush with 4 tablespoons olive oil and roast for 20 to 25 minutes, or until the skins blister and darken.
4. Transfer the peppers to a bowl, cover, and steam for 10 minutes.
5. Peel off the skins and remove the garlic from its peels.

6. Add the roasted peppers, roasted garlic, remaining olive oil, smoked paprika, salt, black pepper, cayenne pepper, tomato paste, plant milk, nutritional yeast, and lemon juice to a blender. Blend until completely smooth.
7. Warm in a saucepan over medium heat for 5 to 7 minutes, stirring occasionally.
8. Adjust salt, lemon, or heat to taste.

Pairs With

Penne, rigatoni, roasted cauliflower, grilled vegetable skewers, couscous bowls, tofu cutlets, quinoa bowls, or warm wraps.

Roasted Red Pepper Sauce II

Creamy, smoky, and naturally sweet, this blended roasted red pepper sauce coats pasta beautifully.

Makes About 4 cups | Prep Time 10 minutes | Cook Time 10 minutes

Ingredients

4 tablespoons olive oil
1½ cups diced onion
6 garlic cloves, minced
3 jars roasted red peppers (12 ounces each), drained
2 cups unsweetened plant milk
8 tablespoons tomato paste
8 tablespoons nutritional yeast
4 tablespoons lemon juice
2 teaspoons smoked paprika
1½ teaspoons fine sea salt
1 teaspoon black pepper
4 tablespoons vegan butter
4 tablespoons cashew cream
2 teaspoons chili flakes
1 cup chopped basil
1 cup chopped parsley
4 cups cooked chickpeas

Directions

1. Warm the olive oil in a saucepan over medium heat. Add the diced onion and cook until softened. Add the garlic and cook for 1 minute.
2. Add the roasted red peppers, plant milk, tomato paste, nutritional yeast, lemon juice, smoked paprika, salt, and black pepper.
3. Simmer for 5 minutes. Transfer to a blender and blend until smooth.
4. Return the sauce to the saucepan and stir in the vegan butter, cashew cream, chili flakes, basil, parsley, and chickpeas. Warm gently and adjust salt or lemon juice to taste.

Pairs With

Pasta, roasted broccoli, sautéed zucchini, chickpeas, tofu, fresh herbs, couscous, quinoa, or grilled vegetables.

Creamy Garlic Tomato Sauce

Creamy, savory, and lightly sweetened, this tomato-based sauce brings together garlic, herbs, and plant milk for a velvety finish ideal for pasta, stuffed shells, lasagna layers, roasted vegetables, or grain bowls.

Makes About 4 cups | Prep Time 10 minutes | Cook Time 15 minutes

Ingredients

4 tablespoons olive oil
1½ cups diced onion
9 garlic cloves, minced
6 cups crushed tomatoes
2 cups unsweetened plant milk
8 tablespoons nutritional yeast
4 tablespoons maple syrup
4 teaspoons onion powder
2 teaspoons garlic powder
1½ teaspoons fine sea salt
1 teaspoon black pepper
4 tablespoons vegan butter
4 tablespoons tahini
2 teaspoons chili flakes
1 cup chopped basil
1 cup chopped oregano
4 cups roasted vegetables (such as zucchini, eggplant, or peppers)

Directions

1. Warm the olive oil in a saucepan over medium heat. Add the diced onion and cook until softened. Add the minced garlic and cook for 1 minute.
2. Add the crushed tomatoes, plant milk, nutritional yeast, maple syrup, onion powder, garlic powder, salt, and black pepper.
3. Simmer for 10 minutes to thicken. Stir in the vegan butter and tahini.
4. Add the chili flakes, basil, oregano, and roasted vegetables.Warm gently and adjust seasoning with additional salt or maple syrup to taste.

Pairs With

Pasta, lasagna layers, stuffed shells, roasted vegetables, tofu, couscous, quinoa, or hearty grain bowls.

Smoky Tomato Paprika Sauce

This robust roasted tomato sauce blends smoked paprika, cumin, roasted garlic, chili flakes, and a touch of tomato paste for a richly seasoned, smoky finish perfect for grain bowls, beans, roasted vegetables, and grilled tofu.

Makes About 4 cups | Prep Time 10 minutes | Cook Time 25 minutes

Ingredients

8 pounds tomatoes, halved

4 small onions, quartered

12 garlic cloves, unpeeled

4 tablespoons olive oil

4 teaspoons smoked paprika

4 roasted red bell peppers, chopped

2 teaspoons ground cumin

2 teaspoons chili flakes

4 teaspoons fine sea salt

2 teaspoons black pepper

4 tablespoons tomato paste

Directions

1. Preheat the oven to 400 degrees. Line a baking sheet with parchment paper. Arrange the tomatoes, onions, and garlic cloves on the sheet.
2. Drizzle with the olive oil and sprinkle with smoked paprika, cumin, chili flakes, salt, and black pepper.
3. Roast for 25 minutes, or until softened and lightly charred.
4. Transfer the roasted vegetables to a saucepan. Remove the garlic skins. Add the tomato paste and the roasted red peppers.
5. Use an immersion blender to blend until smooth or leave slightly chunky.
6. Cook uncovered over medium heat for 5 to 10 minutes to thicken and develop flavor. Adjust salt, pepper, or heat as desired.

Pairs With

Lentil patties, smoky tempeh, roasted potatoes, quinoa bowls, couscous, beans, tofu cutlets, vegetable steaks or grilled mushrooms.

Creamy Smoky Arrabbiata

A rich, velvety spin on classic arrabbiata. Slow-roasted tomatoes, garlic, and chili flakes form the fiery base, while cashew cream adds silkiness and smoked paprika delivers gentle, warm depth.

Makes About 4 cups | Prep Time 10 minutes | Cook Time 30 minutes

Ingredients

8 pounds tomatoes, halved

1 head garlic, cloves separated

1 large onion, quartered

4 tablespoons olive oil

2 teaspoons dried oregano

2 teaspoons dried basil

2 teaspoons crushed red pepper flakes

1 teaspoon fine sea salt

1 teaspoon black pepper

4 tablespoons tomato paste

½ cup vegetable broth

4 tablespoons balsamic vinegar

4 teaspoons maple syrup

1 cup raw cashews, soaked 2+ hours or simmered 10 minutes

1–1½ teaspoons smoked paprika (adjust to taste)

Optional: 1–2 teaspoons liquid smoke for a stronger smoky note

Directions

1. Preheat oven to 400°F and line a baking sheet with parchment.
2. Arrange tomatoes cut-side up; scatter garlic and onion.

3. Drizzle with olive oil and sprinkle with oregano, basil, chili flakes, salt, and pepper.
4. Roast 30 minutes, until tomatoes collapse and edges darken.
5. Transfer roasted vegetables to a saucepan and peel the garlic.
6. Add tomato paste, vegetable broth, balsamic vinegar, and maple syrup.
7. Blend the mixture with the soaked cashews and smoked paprika until completely smooth and creamy.
8. Return to the saucepan and simmer 10 minutes to thicken and meld flavors.
9. Add extra smoked paprika or chili flakes to taste.
10. For a bolder smoky flavor, add 1–2 teaspoons liquid smoke at the end.

Pairs With

Penne, rigatoni, roasted vegetables, tofu steaks, baked potatoes, or grain bowls.

Make It Yours

Stir in roasted red peppers for extra creaminess and sweetness. Add a spoonful of chili crisp for smoky heat. For a lighter version, replace cashews with ½–1 cup unsweetened plant milk.

Mediterranean Olive and Capers Sauce

Briny and herby this Mediterranean-inspired sauce blends roasted tomatoes with kalamata olives, capers, herbs, sun-dried tomatoes, and chili flakes for a savory, tangy, and deeply flavorful finish.

Makes About 4 cups | Prep Time 10 minutes | Cook Time 20 minutes

Ingredients

8 pounds tomatoes, halved

8 garlic cloves, minced

4 tablespoons olive oil

2 cups chopped kalamata olives

8 tablespoons capers, drained

4 tablespoons tomato paste

2 teaspoons dried oregano

2 teaspoons red pepper flakes

2 teaspoons fine sea salt

1 teaspoon black pepper

2 cups chopped fresh basil

2 cups chopped fresh parsley

2 cups chopped sun-dried tomatoes

Directions

1. Preheat the oven to 400 degrees. Line a baking sheet with parchment paper. Arrange the halved tomatoes on the sheet and roast for about 25 minutes, or until softened and slightly caramelized.
2. Warm the olive oil in a large skillet over medium heat. Add the minced garlic and sauté for 1 minute. Add the roasted tomatoes, tomato paste, olives, capers, oregano, red pepper flakes, salt, and black pepper.
3. Add the chopped sun-dried tomatoes and half of the chopped basil and parsley. Blend lightly with an immersion blender — enough to combine but keep texture. Simmer uncovered for 10 to 12 minutes to thicken.
4. Stir in the remaining fresh herbs and adjust seasonings, or heat as needed.

Pairs With

Penne, fusilli, quinoa bowls, roasted eggplant, grilled zucchini, vegan feta, white beans, farro bowls or warm pita dishes.

Tomato White Bean Cream Sauce

Smooth, savory, and protein-rich, this velvety tomato cream sauce blends white beans, balsamic vinegar, roasted vegetables, red pepper flakes, and herbs for a vibrant, versatile finish.

Makes About 4 cups | Prep Time 10 minutes | Cook Time 10 minutes

Ingredients

4 tablespoons olive oil

1½ cups diced onion

8 garlic cloves, minced

6 cups crushed tomatoes

4 cups cooked white beans

2 cups unsweetened plant milk

8 tablespoons nutritional yeast

4 cups roasted vegetables (such as zucchini, peppers, carrots, or eggplant)

4 tablespoons maple syrup

2 teaspoons garlic powder

1½ teaspoons fine sea salt

1 teaspoon black pepper

4 tablespoons balsamic vinegar

4 tablespoons vegan butter

2 teaspoons red pepper flakes

1½ cups chopped basil

Directions

1. Warm the olive oil in a large saucepan over medium heat and add the diced onion. Cook until softened.
2. Add the minced garlic and cook for 1 minute. Add the crushed tomatoes, white beans, plant milk, nutritional yeast, maple syrup, garlic powder, salt, and black pepper.
3. Simmer for 5 minutes. Transfer the mixture to a blender and blend until completely smooth.
4. Return the sauce to the saucepan and stir in the balsamic vinegar, vegan butter, red pepper flakes, basil, and roasted vegetables. Warm gently, then taste and adjust salt, lemon, or pepper.

Fire Roasted Tomato Basil Sauce

Smoky, bright, and full of depth, this fire-roasted tomato sauce blends garlic, basil, smoked paprika, balsamic vinegar, and vegan butter into a velvety, flavorful finish perfect for pasta, casseroles, stews, and lasagna.

Makes About 4 cups | Prep Time 10 minutes | Cook Time 15 minutes

Ingredients

4 tablespoons olive oil

1½ cups diced onion

9 garlic cloves, minced

4 cans fire-roasted diced tomatoes (14 ounces each)

2 cups unsweetened plant milk or vegetable broth

4 tablespoons tomato paste

4 tablespoons balsamic vinegar

4 teaspoons dried basil

2 teaspoons smoked paprika

1½ teaspoons fine sea salt

1 teaspoon black pepper

4 tablespoons vegan butter

1 cup chopped fresh basil

4 tablespoons nutritional yeast

2 teaspoons red pepper flakes

4 cups roasted vegetables (such as zucchini, bell peppers, or eggplant)

4 cups cooked white beans

Directions

1. Warm the olive oil in a saucepan over medium heat.
2. Add the diced onion and cook until softened.

3. Add the garlic and cook for 1 minute.
4. Add the fire-roasted tomatoes, plant milk or broth, tomato paste, balsamic vinegar, dried basil, smoked paprika, salt, and black pepper.
5. Simmer for 10 to 12 minutes.
6. Stir in the vegan butter, fresh basil, nutritional yeast, red pepper flakes, roasted vegetables, and white beans.
7. Warm gently and adjust seasoning to taste.

Pairs With

Pasta, lasagna layers, stuffed shells, gnocchi, casseroles, roasted vegetables, polenta, soups or grain bowls.

3. Creamy Sauces and Cashew Blends

Silky, satisfying, and full of body — these cashew-based sauces deliver comfort without heaviness. Whether stirred into pasta, spooned over roasted vegetables, or used as a base for soups and casseroles, cashews bring rich creaminess that balances beautifully with herbs, citrus, or spice.

Classic Cashew Cream Sauce
Mushroom Cashew Cream Sauce
Garlic Tahini Cashew Cream Sauce
Coconut Curry Cashew Sauce
Lemon Dill Cashew Sauce
Creamy Dill Pasta Sauce
White Bean Alfredo Sauce
Creamy Cold Noodle Sauce
Lemon Pasta Salad Sauce
Miso Lemon Pasta Sauce
Cashew Cauliflower Alfredo
Lemon Caper Pasta Sauce
Walnut Mushroom Bolognese
Lemon Herb Orzo Sauce
Vegetable 'Cream' Sauce Base
Creamy Spinach Pasta Sauce
Caramelized Onion Pasta Sauce
Sweet Corn Pasta Sauce
Green Goddess Pasta Sauce
Butternut or Pumpkin Cream Sauce
Creamy Artichoke Pasta Sauce
Lemon Parsley 'Butter' Sauce
Garlic White Bean 'Scampi' Sauce
Cashew Pesto Cream Sauce
Roasted Garlic Alfredo
Creamy Sunflower Seed Pasta Sauce
Lemon Tahini Pasta Sauce
Mushroom Marsala Pasta Sauce
Caramelized Fennel Pasta Sauce
Zesty Roasted Lemon Sauce
Cashew 'Ricotta' Pasta Sauce
Creamy Garlic Herb Mushroom Sauce
Bruschetta Pasta Sauce

Classic Cashew Cream Sauce

A silky, all-purpose staple that brings richness to everything from pasta and soups to roasted vegetables and grain bowls.

Makes About 4 cups | Prep Time 5 minutes | Soak Time 30 minutes | Cook Time 5 minutes

Ingredients

2 cups raw cashews
3½ cups hot water
1 small garlic clove
2 tablespoons lemon juice
1 teaspoon fine sea salt
½ teaspoon black pepper
3 tablespoons nutritional yeast
1 teaspoon maple syrup
1 pinch smoked paprika
1 pinch cayenne pepper

Directions

1. Soak the cashews in hot water for 30 minutes and drain.
2. Add the soaked cashews, garlic, lemon juice, salt, pepper, nutritional yeast, maple syrup, smoked paprika, cayenne pepper, and 3 cups of the hot water to a blender.
3. Blend until completely smooth.
4. Add the remaining hot water as needed to reach a smooth, pourable consistency.
5. Pour the mixture into a saucepan and warm gently for 3 to 5 minutes, stirring occasionally, until slightly thickened.

Pairs With

Pasta, roasted broccoli, steamed greens, grain bowls, roasted potatoes, casseroles, or creamy soups.

Mushroom Cashew Cream Sauce

Earthy mushrooms blend seamlessly into a rich cashew base, creating an umami-packed sauce that is comforting, savory and perfect for coating pasta.

Makes About 4 cups | Prep Time 10 minutes | Cook Time 15 minutes

Ingredients

1 tablespoon olive oil

2 cups sliced cremini or button mushrooms

1 small shallot, minced

2 garlic cloves, minced

2 cups raw cashews, soaked for 30 minutes

3½ cups hot water

2 tablespoons lemon juice

1 teaspoon fine sea salt

½ teaspoon black pepper

2 tablespoons tomato paste

1 pinch crushed red pepper

1 pinch smoked paprika

Directions

1. Heat the olive oil in a skillet over medium heat. Add the mushrooms and cook for 5 to 6 minutes until tender and lightly browned.
2. Add the shallot and garlic and cook for 2 more minutes.
3. Add the cooked mixture, soaked cashews, hot water, lemon juice, salt, black pepper, tomato paste, crushed red pepper, and smoked paprika to a blender.
4. Blend until completely smooth.
5. Pour the sauce into a saucepan and warm over low heat for 5 minutes, stirring occasionally, until thickened.

Pairs With

Pasta, baked tempeh, sautéed kale, mashed potatoes, roasted vegetables, or grain bowls.

Garlic Tahini Cashew Cream Sauce

Cashew cream blends with tahini, garlic, and warm spices to create a rich, silky sauce perfect for drizzling, tossing, or dipping.

Makes About 4 cups | Prep Time 10 minutes | Cook Time 5 minutes

Ingredients

2 cups raw cashews, soaked for 30 minutes

1 cup tahini

4 garlic cloves

4 tablespoons lemon juice

1 teaspoon fine sea salt

1 teaspoon ground cumin

4 cups warm water

4 tablespoons olive oil

4 tablespoons maple syrup

1 pinch cayenne pepper

1 tablespoon harissa paste

Directions

1. Drain the soaked cashews. Add the cashews, tahini, garlic, lemon juice, salt, cumin, warm water, olive oil, maple syrup, cayenne pepper, and harissa paste to a blender. Blend until completely smooth and creamy.
2. Pour the sauce into a small saucepan and warm gently for 3 to 5 minutes, stirring constantly, until slightly thickened. Add more warm water if a thinner, drizzle-style consistency is desired.

Pairs With

Falafel, roasted cauliflower, grain bowls, wraps, roasted potatoes, or sautéed greens.

Coconut Curry Cashew Sauce

A fragrant blend of cashews, coconut milk, warm curry spices, lime, and cilantro creates a creamy, aromatic sauce that elevates pasta, rice, tofu, and vegetables.

Makes About 4 cups | Prep Time 10 minutes | Cook Time 15 minutes

Ingredients

2 teaspoons coconut oil
2 small onions, finely chopped
4 garlic cloves, minced
2 teaspoons grated fresh ginger
4 tablespoons curry powder
2 cups raw cashews, soaked 30 minutes
2 cans light coconut milk
1½ teaspoons fine sea salt
2 tablespoons tomato paste
4 tablespoons lime juice
½ cup chopped fresh cilantro
1 pinch cayenne pepper

Directions

1. Heat the coconut oil in a saucepan over medium heat.
2. Add the onions, garlic, and ginger and cook for 5 minutes until fragrant and softened.
3. Add the curry powder and cayenne pepper and cook for 1 minute to toast the spices.
4. Add the soaked cashews, coconut milk, tomato paste, salt, lime juice, and cilantro to the blender along with the cooked mixture.
5. Blend until completely smooth.
6. Return the sauce to the saucepan and cook over medium heat for 5 to 7 minutes, stirring occasionally, until thickened and creamy.

Pairs With

Steamed rice, roasted chickpeas, grilled tofu, sautéed vegetables, grain bowls, or rice noodles.

Lemon Dill Cashew Sauce

Bright, tangy, and herby, this creamy lemon-dill cashew sauce adds a citrus layer to pasta, grain bowls, wraps, roasted vegetables, and spring dishes.

Makes About 4 cups | Prep Time 10 minutes | Cook Time 5 minutes

Ingredients

2 cups raw cashews, soaked for 30 minutes

3½ cups hot water

6 tablespoons lemon juice

4 tablespoons olive oil

½ cup chopped fresh dill

1½ teaspoons fine sea salt

½ teaspoon black pepper

4 garlic cloves

2 teaspoons Dijon mustard

4 tablespoons nutritional yeast

1 pinch crushed red pepper flakes

Directions

1. Drain the soaked cashews. Add the cashews, hot water, lemon juice, olive oil, dill, salt, black pepper, garlic, Dijon mustard, nutritional yeast, and crushed red pepper flakes to a blender.
2. Blend until completely smooth.
3. Pour the sauce into a small saucepan and warm gently over low heat for 3 to 5 minutes, stirring occasionally, until slightly thickened.

Pairs With

Roasted potatoes, grilled tempeh, quinoa bowls, steamed asparagus, pasta, roasted carrots, or baked tofu.

Creamy Dill Pasta Sauce

Creamy, savory, lemony, and herby, this sauce blends cashews, plant milk, and fresh dill into a bright, velvety finish reminiscent of a lighter Alfredo. It coats pasta beautifully without feeling heavy.

Makes About 4 cups | Prep Time 10 minutes | Cook Time 10 minutes

Ingredients

4 tablespoons olive oil

1½ cups diced onion

6 garlic cloves, minced

4 cups unsweetened plain plant milk

1½ cups raw cashews, soaked in hot water for 10 minutes

6 tablespoons lemon juice

4 tablespoons white wine vinegar

4 tablespoons nutritional yeast

1 cup chopped fresh dill

2 teaspoons garlic powder

2 teaspoons onion powder

1½ teaspoons fine sea salt

1 teaspoon black pepper

4 tablespoons vegan butter

4 tablespoons tahini

Zest of 2 lemons

2 handfuls baby spinach

Directions

1. Warm the olive oil in a large saucepan over medium heat.
2. Add the diced onion and cook until softened.

3. Add the garlic and cook for 1 minute.
4. Add the plant milk, soaked cashews, lemon juice, white wine vinegar, nutritional yeast, garlic powder, onion powder, salt, and black pepper.
5. Simmer for 5 minutes to fully soften the cashews.
6. Transfer the mixture to a blender.
7. Add the lemon zest and baby spinach, then blend until completely smooth.
8. Return the blended sauce to the saucepan and stir in the fresh dill, vegan butter, and tahini.
9. Warm gently over low heat for 2 to 3 minutes, stirring occasionally.
10. Adjust lemon juice, salt, or dill to taste before serving.

Pairs With

Linguine, fettuccine, or penne; roasted asparagus, carrots, broccoli, or zucchini; chickpeas or white beans; baked potatoes; pan-seared tofu cutlets; crispy baked tofu; or warm grain bowls.

White Bean Alfredo Sauce

Creamy, smooth, and savory, this Alfredo-style sauce blends white beans, cashews, tahini, and miso into a silky finish that coats pasta beautifully.

Makes About 4 cups | Prep Time 10 minutes | Cook Time 10 minutes

Ingredients

4 tablespoons olive oil
1½ cups diced onion
6 garlic cloves, minced
4 cups cooked cannellini or navy beans
4 cups unsweetened plain plant milk
6 tablespoons nutritional yeast
4 tablespoons lemon juice
2 teaspoons garlic powder
2 teaspoons onion powder
1½ teaspoons fine sea salt
1 teaspoon black pepper
1 cup soaked cashews
4 tablespoons tahini
4 tablespoons vegan butter
2 teaspoons white miso paste
1 pinch nutmeg

Directions

1. Warm the olive oil in a large saucepan over medium heat.
2. Add the diced onion and cook until softened. Add the garlic and cook for 1 minute. Add the white beans, plant milk, nutritional yeast, lemon juice, garlic powder, onion powder, salt, and black pepper.
3. Add the soaked cashews and simmer for 5 minutes. Transfer the mixture to a blender and blend until completely smooth. Return the sauce to the saucepan. Stir in the tahini, vegan butter, miso paste, and nutmeg.
4. Warm gently for 2 to 3 minutes, stirring occasionally. Adjust lemon juice, salt, or pepper to taste before serving.

Pairs With

Fettuccine, penne, sautéed mushrooms, steamed broccoli, roasted cauliflower, gnocchi, or pan-seared tofu.

Creamy Cold Noodle Sauce

Smooth, velvety, and refreshing, this chilled sauce blends tahini, cashews, miso, peanut butter, and aromatics for a finish that clings beautifully to cold noodles.

Makes About 4 cups | Prep Time 10 minutes | Cook Time 5 minutes

Ingredients

1 cup tahini
1 cup raw cashews*
8 tablespoons soy sauce or tamari
4 tablespoons rice vinegar
4 tablespoons lime juice
4 tablespoons maple syrup
4 tablespoons sesame oil
4 teaspoons grated fresh ginger
4 garlic cloves, grated
2 cups water
4 teaspoons white miso paste
4 tablespoons creamy peanut butter
1 teaspoon chili flakes
1 tablespoon chili crisp
1 cup finely diced cucumber
1 cup shredded carrots
1 cup sliced scallions
4 tablespoons sesame seeds

* soaked in hot water for 10 minutes

Directions

1. Add the soaked cashews, tahini, soy sauce or tamari, rice vinegar, lime juice, maple syrup, sesame oil, ginger, garlic, miso paste, peanut butter, and 1½ cups of the water to a blender. Blend until completely smooth.
2. Add more of the remaining water until the sauce reaches a smooth, pourable cold-noodle consistency. Stir in the chili flakes and chili crisp.
3. Fold in the cucumber, carrots, scallions, and sesame seeds, or mix them into the noodle bowl after tossing the noodles with the sauce. Adjust soy sauce, lime juice, or maple syrup to taste.

Pairs With - Cold soba noodles, udon, rice noodles, chilled spaghetti, grain bowls, shredded cabbage salads, tofu or summer vegetable bowls.

Lemon Pasta Salad Sauce

Bright, zesty, and refreshing, this lemony sauce is designed specifically for cold pasta salads. It stays light, balanced, and flavorful without weighing down vegetables, beans, tof, or greens.

Makes About 4 cups | Prep Time 10 minutes | Cook Time None

Ingredients

1 cup olive oil
12 tablespoons lemon juice
4 tablespoons apple cider vinegar
4 tablespoons white wine vinegar
4 tablespoons maple syrup
4 tablespoons Dijon mustard
4 garlic cloves, grated
2 teaspoons garlic powder
1½ teaspoons fine sea salt
1 teaspoon black pepper
Zest of 4 lemons
4 tablespoons vegan yogurt
4 tablespoons parsley, finely chopped
4 tablespoons chives, finely chopped
4 tablespoons capers
4 tablespoons pickle brine
2 teaspoons red pepper flakes
½ cup water

Directions

1. Add the olive oil, lemon juice, apple cider vinegar, white wine vinegar, maple syrup, Dijon mustard, grated garlic, garlic powder, salt, black pepper, lemon zest, vegan yogurt, parsley, chives, capers, pickle brine, and red pepper flakes to a bowl or large jar.
2. Whisk or shake vigorously until fully emulsified.
3. Add the water to lighten the dressing and whisk again.
4. Taste and adjust lemon, salt, or vinegar as needed.

Pairs With

Rotini, bowties, penne, or orzo; cherry tomatoes, cucumbers, olives, chickpeas, arugula, white beans, tofu cubes, and grain bowls.

Miso Lemon Pasta Sauce

Bright, savory, and umami-rich, this lemon–miso sauce creates a light, glossy coating that pairs beautifully with pasta, grain bowls tofu and more.

Makes About 4 cups | Prep Time 10 minutes | Cook Time 5 minutes

Ingredients

8 tablespoons olive oil
8 garlic cloves, minced
4 cups unsweetened plant milk
4 tablespoons white miso paste
8 tablespoons lemon juice
4 tablespoons apple cider vinegar
4 tablespoons nutritional yeast
2 teaspoons garlic powder
1½ teaspoons fine sea salt
1 teaspoon black pepper
Zest of 4 lemons
4 tablespoons vegan butter
4 tablespoons tahini
2 cups peas
4 cups baby spinach
2 cups sautéed mushrooms
2 teaspoons red pepper flakes

Directions

1. Warm the olive oil in a saucepan over medium heat. Add the minced garlic and cook until fragrant. Add the plant milk, miso paste, lemon juice, apple cider vinegar, nutritional yeast, garlic powder, salt, and black pepper.
2. Whisk until the miso dissolves completely. Simmer for 2 to 3 minutes to thicken slightly. Add the lemon zest, vegan butter, tahini, red pepper flakes, peas, spinach, and sautéed mushrooms.
3. Warm gently until the spinach wilts and the vegetables heat through. Adjust lemon, salt, or pepper to taste before serving.

Pairs With

Pasta, white beans, tofu, sautéed mushrooms, peas, asparagus, spinach, roasted vegetables, or grain-based salads.

Cashew Cauliflower Alfredo

Creamy, silky, and surprisingly light, this creation blends steamed cauliflower, cashews, nutmeg, roasted garlic, tahini, and vegan butter into a smooth sauce.

Makes About 4 cups | Prep Time 10 minutes | Cook Time 15 minutes

Ingredients

6 cups cauliflower florets
1½ cups raw cashews*
4 tablespoons olive oil
1½ cups diced onion
6 garlic cloves, minced
4 cups unsweetened plant milk
6 tablespoons nutritional yeast
6 tablespoons lemon juice
2 teaspoons garlic powder
2 teaspoons onion powder
1½ teaspoons fine sea salt
1 teaspoon black pepper
4 tablespoons vegan butter
4 tablespoons tahini
1 teaspoon ground nutmeg
4 tablespoons roasted garlic
2 cups baby spinach
2 cups peas

* soaked in hot water for 10 minutes

Directions

1. Steam the cauliflower until very soft.
2. Warm the olive oil in a large saucepan over medium heat. Add the diced onion and cook until softened.
3. Add the minced garlic and cook for 1 minute.
4. Add the steamed cauliflower, soaked cashews, plant milk, nutritional yeast, lemon juice, garlic powder, onion powder, salt, black pepper, nutmeg, and roasted garlic.
5. Simmer for 5 minutes.

6. Transfer the mixture to a blender and blend until completely smooth. Return the sauce to the saucepan and stir in the vegan butter and tahini.
7. Add the baby spinach and peas and warm gently until the spinach wilts.
8. Adjust seasoning with additional salt, lemon juice, or pepper to taste.

Pairs With

Fettuccine, linguine, penne, roasted broccoli, wilted spinach, peas, white beans, tofu, potato gnocchi, or roasted vegetables.

Lemon Caper Pasta Sauce

Tangy, briny, and vibrant, this lemon–caper sauce brings a piccata-style brightness to pasta, vegetables, tofu, beans, and grain bowls.

Makes About 4 cups | Prep Time 10 minutes | Cook Time 5 minutes

Ingredients

1 cup olive oil

12 garlic cloves, minced

12 tablespoons lemon juice

4 tablespoons white wine vinegar

8 tablespoons chopped capers

4 tablespoons Dijon mustard

2 teaspoons garlic powder

1 cup water

1 teaspoon fine sea salt

1 teaspoon black pepper

Zest of 4 lemons

2 teaspoons chili flakes

4 tablespoons vegan butter

1 cup chopped parsley

1 cup chopped basil

2 cups sautéed mushrooms

4 cups cooked white beans

Directions

1. Warm the olive oil in a saucepan over medium heat. Add the garlic and cook until fragrant.
2. Add the lemon juice, white wine vinegar, capers, Dijon mustard, garlic powder, water, salt, and black pepper.
3. Simmer for 2 to 3 minutes. Add the lemon zest and vegan butter and whisk until melted. Stir in the chili flakes, parsley, basil, mushrooms, and white beans. Warm gently for 1 to 2 minutes. Adjust lemon or salt to taste.

Pairs With

Pasta, roasted vegetables, pan-seared tofu, sautéed mushrooms, white beans, couscous, quinoa bowls, or roasted broccoli.

Walnut Mushroom Bolognese

Hearty, savory, and deeply flavorful, this plant-based bolognese blends mushrooms, walnuts, aromatic vegetables, tomato, miso, and balsamic for a rich, slow-simmered texture perfect for pasta, polenta, and baked dishes.

Makes About 4 cups | Prep Time 15 minutes | Cook Time 25 minutes

Ingredients

4 tablespoons olive oil
4 cups finely chopped mushrooms
2 cups diced onion
4 medium carrots, finely diced
8 garlic cloves, minced
2 cups finely chopped walnuts
4 cups crushed tomatoes
2 cups vegetable broth
8 tablespoons tomato paste
4 tablespoons soy sauce or tamari
4 teaspoons smoked paprika
2 teaspoons garlic powder
1½ teaspoons fine sea salt
1 teaspoon black pepper
4 teaspoons balsamic vinegar
4 teaspoons white miso paste
2 cups cooked lentils
4 cups chopped spinach or kale
2 teaspoons chili flakes

Directions

1. Warm the olive oil in a large skillet over medium heat. Add the mushrooms, onion and carrot. Sauté until softened.
2. Add the garlic and cook for 1 minute. Add the walnuts, crushed tomatoes, vegetable broth, tomato paste, soy sauce, smoked paprika, garlic powder, salt, and black pepper.
3. Simmer for 15 to 20 minutes until thickened. Stir in the balsamic vinegar, miso paste, lentils, and spinach or kale. Warm until the greens wilt. Add chili flakes and adjust seasoning to taste.

Pairs With - Spaghetti, linguine, rigatoni, polenta, lasagna layers, baked pasta dishes, roasted vegetables, or garlic bread.

Lemon Herb Orzo Sauce

Light, bright, and herby, this lemony sauce is perfect for warm or cold orzo salads. It stays clean and refreshing while still coating pasta thoroughly.

Makes About 4 cups | Prep Time 10 minutes | Cook Time None

Ingredients

1 cup olive oil
12 tablespoons lemon juice
4 tablespoons white wine vinegar
4 tablespoons Dijon mustard
4 tablespoons maple syrup
4 garlic cloves, grated
1 cup chopped fresh parsley
1 cup chopped fresh basil
Zest of 4 lemons
4 tablespoons vegan yogurt
1½ teaspoons fine sea salt
1 teaspoon black pepper
1 cup capers
2 cups halved cherry tomatoes
2 cups sliced olives
4 cups cooked white beans or chickpeas, canned or cooked

Directions

1. Add the olive oil, lemon juice, white wine vinegar, Dijon mustard, maple syrup, grated garlic, chopped parsley, chopped basil, lemon zest, vegan yogurt, salt, and black pepper to a large bowl or jar.
2. Whisk or shake vigorously until emulsified.
3. Stir in the capers, cherry tomatoes, olives, and chickpeas or white beans.
4. Adjust lemon or salt to taste.

Pairs With

Orzo salads (warm or cold), couscous bowls, quinoa salads, roasted vegetables, cherry tomatoes, tofu, white beans, or Mediterranean-style bowls.

Vegetable "Cream Sauce" Base

Light and velvety, this blended vegetable-based sauce creates a versatile foundation for many pasta dishes, casseroles, grain bowls, or soups. Its clean flavor is designed to be adapted any direction you like.

Makes About 4 cups | Prep Time 10 minutes | Cook Time 15 minutes

Ingredients

6 cups cauliflower florets

1½ cups diced onion

2 medium carrots, chopped

2 sticks celery, chopped

6 garlic cloves

4 cups vegetable broth

1½ cups soaked cashews

8 tablespoons nutritional yeast

4 tablespoons lemon juice

2 teaspoons garlic powder

1½ teaspoons fine sea salt

1 teaspoon black pepper

2 teaspoons white miso paste

1 cup chopped parsley

1 cup chopped basil

1 tablespoon chopped thyme

8 tablespoons tomato paste

4 tablespoons vegan butter

4 tablespoons roasted garlic

Directions

1. Add the cauliflower, onion, carrots, celery, garlic, and vegetable broth to a large saucepan. Bring to a simmer and cook until all vegetables are soft.
2. Add the soaked cashews, nutritional yeast, lemon juice, garlic powder, salt, black pepper, miso paste, parsley, basil, thyme, tomato paste, vegan butter, and roasted garlic.
3. Transfer everything to a blender and blend until completely smooth. Return the sauce to the saucepan and warm gently. Adjust seasoning with additional salt, lemon juice, or pepper to taste.

Pairs With - Pasta, casseroles, macaroni-style bakes, creamy soups, roasted vegetables, gnocchi, or grain bowls.

Creamy Spinach Pasta Sauce

Silky, vibrant, and naturally green, this creamy spinach sauce combines cashews, lemon, herbs, and aromatics for a light, clean flavor. .

Makes About 4 cups | Prep Time 10 minutes | Cook Time 10 minutes

Ingredients

4 tablespoons olive oil
1½ cups diced onion
6 garlic cloves, minced
8 cups fresh spinach, packed
4 cups unsweetened plant milk
1½ cups raw cashews *
8 tablespoons nutritional yeast
4 tablespoons lemon juice
2 teaspoons garlic powder
* soaked in hot water for 10 minutes

1½ teaspoons fine sea salt
1 teaspoon black pepper
Zest of 2 lemons
1 cup chopped basil
1 cup chopped parsley
2 teaspoons chili flakes
2 cups peas
2 cups chopped artichoke hearts

Directions

1. Warm the olive oil in a large saucepan over medium heat. Add the diced onion and cook until softened.
2. Add the garlic and cook for 1 minute. Add the spinach and cook until wilted. Add the plant milk, soaked cashews, nutritional yeast, lemon juice, garlic powder, salt, and black pepper.
3. Simmer for 5 minutes. Transfer the mixture to a blender and add the lemon zest, basil, parsley, chili flakes, peas, and artichokes. Blend until completely smooth. Return the sauce to the saucepan and warm gently. Adjust lemon, salt, or pepper to taste.

Pairs With - Pasta, gnocchi, roasted vegetables, peas, artichokes, tofu, white beans, or grain bowls.

Caramelized Onion Pasta Sauce

Sweet, savory, and deeply flavored, this velvety sauce is built on slow-caramelized onions blended with plant milk, herbs, vinegar, and mushrooms for richness and depth.

Makes About 4 cups | Prep Time 15 minutes | Cook Time 20 minutes

Ingredients

4 tablespoons olive oil

8 medium onions, thinly sliced

8 garlic cloves, minced

4 cups unsweetened plant milk

8 tablespoons balsamic vinegar

4 tablespoons nutritional yeast

1 teaspoon black pepper

4 tablespoons vegan butter

2 tablespoons chopped rosemary

2 tablespoons chopped thyme

4 cups sliced mushrooms

2 cups vegetable broth

1½ teaspoons fine sea salt

Directions

1. Warm the olive oil in a wide pan over medium heat. Add the sliced onions and cook until deeply golden and caramelized.
2. Add the garlic and cook for 1 minute. Add the mushrooms and cook until softened. Add the plant milk, vinegar, nutritional yeast, rosemary, thyme, salt, black pepper, and vegetable broth.
3. Simmer for 5 minutes.
4. Transfer the mixture to a blender and blend until completely smooth. Return the sauce to the pan and stir in the vegan butter. Warm gently and adjust salt or vinegar to taste.

Pairs With

Pasta, gnocchi, mashed potatoes, polenta, roasted mushrooms, green beans, grilled tofu or grain bowls.

Sweet Corn Pasta Sauce

Creamy, naturally sweet, and summery, this corn-based pasta sauce blends aromatics, basil, roasted peppers, and a hint of lemon for a velvety finish that pairs beautifully with grilled vegetables and black pepper.

Makes About 4 cups | Prep Time 10 minutes | Cook Time 10 minutes

Ingredients

4 tablespoons olive oil

1½ cups diced onion

8 cups corn kernels (fresh or frozen)

4 cups unsweetened plant milk

4 tablespoons lemon juice

4 tablespoons nutritional yeast

2 teaspoons garlic powder

1½ teaspoons fine sea salt

1 teaspoon black pepper

4 tablespoons vegan butter

1½ cups soaked cashews

2 cups chopped fresh basil

2 cups chopped roasted red peppers

2 teaspoons chili flakes

Directions

1. Warm the olive oil in a large saucepan over medium heat. Add the diced onion and cook until softened. Add the corn kernels and cook for 3 minutes.

2. Add the plant milk, lemon juice, nutritional yeast, garlic powder, salt, and pepper. Add the soaked cashews, basil, roasted red peppers, and chili flakes.

3. Simmer for 5 minutes.

4. Transfer the mixture to a blender and blend until completely smooth. Return the sauce to the saucepan and stir in the vegan butter. Warm gently and adjust lemon, salt, or pepper to taste.

Pairs With - Pasta, grilled zucchini, roasted peppers, basil, black pepper, tofu, gnocchi or summer vegetable bowls.

Green Goddess Pasta Sauce

Bright, herbal, creamy, and dairy-free, this vibrant green sauce blends avocado, herbs, yogurt, spinach, mint, capers, and jalapeño for a fresh, flavorful finish that works beautifully with warm pasta, pasta salads, bowls, or roasted vegetables.

Makes About 4 cups | Prep Time 10 minutes | Cook Time None

Ingredients

4 ripe avocados
4 cups plain unsweetened vegan yogurt or silken tofu
1 cup lemon juice
4 garlic cloves
1 cup fresh parsley
1 cup fresh basil
8 tablespoons fresh chives
4 tablespoons olive oil
1½ teaspoons fine sea salt
1 teaspoon black pepper
4 tablespoons white wine vinegar
4 handfuls fresh spinach
½ cup fresh mint leaves
½ cup capers
1 jalapeño, seeds removed for mild heat or left in for spicy heat

Directions

1. Add the avocados, vegan yogurt or tofu, lemon juice, garlic, parsley, basil, chives, olive oil, salt, and black pepper to a blender.
2. Add the white wine vinegar, spinach, mint, capers and jalapeño.
3. Blend until completely smooth and vibrant green. Taste and adjust lemon juice, salt, or pepper as needed.

Pairs With

Warm pasta bowls, cold pasta salads, quinoa bowls, roasted potatoes, asparagus, broccoli, tofu, grain bowls, or roasted summer vegetables.

Butternut or Pumpkin Cream Sauce

Creamy, savory, lightly sweet, and ultra-smooth, this blended squash-based sauce features sage, smoked paprika, roasted garlic, tahini, and cashews for depth and richness.

Makes About 4 cups | Prep Time 10 minutes | Cook Time 15 minutes

Ingredients

4 cups cooked butternut squash or pumpkin purée
4 tablespoons olive oil
1½ cups diced onion
6 garlic cloves, minced
4 cups vegetable broth
2 cups unsweetened plant milk
8 tablespoons nutritional yeast
4 tablespoons lemon juice
2 teaspoons garlic powder
1½ teaspoons fine sea salt
1 teaspoon black pepper
4 tablespoons vegan butter
4 tablespoons tahini
1½ cups soaked cashews
8 tablespoons roasted garlic
2 teaspoons smoked paprika
2 tablespoons chopped fresh sage
4 tablespoons apple cider vinegar

Directions

1. Warm the olive oil in a large saucepan over medium heat. Add the diced onion and cook until softened.
2. Add the minced garlic. Cook for 1 minute.
3. Add the cooked butternut squash or pumpkin, vegetable broth, plant milk, nutritional yeast, lemon juice, garlic powder, salt, black pepper, roasted garlic, smoked paprika, sage, and vinegar.
4. Add the soaked cashews and simmer for 5 to 7 minutes to meld flavors.
5. Transfer the mixture to a blender and blend until completely smooth.
6. Return the sauce to the saucepan and stir in the vegan butter and tahini.

7. Warm gently over low heat and adjust seasoning with additional salt, pepper, or lemon juice to taste.

Pairs With

Pasta, gnocchi, roasted vegetables, sautéed greens, tofu, white beans, farro, quinoa, baked casseroles, or autumn-inspired bowls.

Creamy Artichoke Pasta Sauce

Smooth, tangy, and savory, this Mediterranean-inspired sauce blends artichokes, cashews, capers, herbs, and lemon into a velvety finish.

Makes About 4 cups | Prep Time 10 minutes | Cook Time 10 minutes

Ingredients

4 tablespoons olive oil
1½ cups diced onion
6 garlic cloves, minced
4 cans artichoke hearts (14 ounces each), drained
4 cups unsweetened plant milk
4 tablespoons nutritional yeast
4 tablespoons lemon juice
2 teaspoons garlic powder
1½ teaspoons fine sea salt
1 teaspoon black pepper
4 tablespoons vegan butter
1½ cups soaked cashews
1 cup capers
1 cup chopped olives
1 cup chopped basil
1 cup chopped parsley
2 cups chopped roasted red peppers
2 cups fresh spinach
2 cups peas

Directions

1. Warm the olive oil in a large saucepan over medium heat. Add the diced onion and cook until softened. Add the garlic and cook for 1 minute. Add the artichoke hearts, plant milk, nutritional yeast, lemon juice, garlic powder, salt, and black pepper.

2. Add the soaked cashews, capers, olives, basil, parsley, roasted red peppers, spinach, and peas. Simmer for 5 minutes. Transfer the mixture to a blender and blend until completely smooth.

3. Return the sauce to the saucepan and stir in the vegan butter. Warm gently and adjust salt or lemon juice to taste.

Pairs With - Pasta, gnocchi, orzo, couscous, roasted vegetables, sautéed greens, white beans, polenta, or Mediterranean-style bowls.

Lemon Parsley 'Butter' Sauce

Bright, buttery, and herby, this lemon–parsley sauce blends vegan butter, garlic, capers, lemon zest, and chili flakes into a rich yet vibrant finish perfect for pasta, gnocchi, vegetables, or tofu.

Makes About 4 cups | Prep Time 10 minutes | Cook Time 5 minutes

Ingredients

1½ cups vegan butter

½ cup olive oil

12 garlic cloves, minced

12 tablespoons lemon juice

1 cup vegetable stock

1 cup chopped fresh parsley

1½ teaspoons fine sea salt

1 teaspoon black pepper

Zest of 4 lemons

2 teaspoons chili flakes

1½ cups capers

Directions

1. Add the vegan butter and olive oil to a saucepan over medium heat. Add the minced garlic and cook until fragrant. Add the lemon juice, vegetable stock, parsley, salt, and black pepper.
2. Warm gently for 1 to 2 minutes. Stir in the lemon zest, chili flakes, and capers. Adjust salt, lemon juice, or pepper to taste.

Pairs With

Pasta, gnocchi, roasted potatoes, asparagus, sautéed greens, tofu cutlets, white beans, or grilled vegetables.

Garlic White Bean 'Scampi' Sauce

Inspired by classic scampi flavors, this silky, dairy-free sauce blends white beans with garlic, lemon, vegan butter, and herbs for a bright, savory, luxurious finish.

Makes about 4 cups | Prep Time 10 minutes | Cook Time 10 minutes

Ingredients

4 tablespoons olive oil
16 garlic cloves, minced
4 cups cooked white beans
2 cups vegetable broth
1¼ cups lemon juice
4 tablespoons vegan butter
4 tablespoons nutritional yeast
1½ teaspoons fine sea salt
1 teaspoon black pepper
Zest of 4 lemons
2 teaspoons chili flakes
1 cup chopped parsley
4 cups roasted mushrooms
1 teaspoon maple syrup (optional)

Directions

1. Warm the olive oil in a large saucepan over medium heat.
2. Add the minced garlic and cook until fragrant.
3. Add the white beans, vegetable broth, lemon juice, vegan butter, nutritional yeast, salt, and black pepper.
4. Simmer for 5 minutes.
5. Transfer the mixture to a blender and blend until completely smooth.
6. Return the sauce to the pan. Stir in the lemon zest, chili flakes, parsley, roasted mushrooms and maple syrup, if using.
7. Warm until heated through. Serve with pasta, grains, vegetables, or tofu.

Pairs With - Pasta, roasted mushrooms, asparagus, sautéed greens, tofu cutlets, polenta, or white beans.

Cashew Pesto Cream Sauce

Creamy, bright, and aromatic, this basil-flavored sauce blends cashews, spinach, roasted tomatoes, and lemon for a silky pesto-style cream perfect for pasta, gnocchi, grains, and roasted vegetables.

Makes About 4 cups | Prep Time 10 minutes | Cook Time 5 minutes

Ingredients

4 cups unsweetened plant milk
1½ cups raw cashews *
4 cups fresh basil leaves, packed
8 tablespoons lemon juice
8 tablespoons nutritional yeast
8 garlic cloves
4 tablespoons olive oil
1½ teaspoons fine sea salt
1 teaspoon black pepper
4 tablespoons vegan butter
Zest of 2 lemons
4 cups fresh spinach
2 teaspoons chili flakes
4 cups roasted cherry tomatoes

* soaked in hot water for 10 minutes

Directions

1. Add the plant milk, soaked cashews, basil, lemon juice, nutritional yeast, garlic, olive oil, salt, and black pepper to a blender.
2. Add the spinach, lemon zest, chili flakes, and roasted cherry tomatoes.
3. Blend until completely smooth and vibrant green.
4. Pour the sauce into a saucepan and warm gently over low heat, stirring often. Avoid boiling to preserve the green color.
5. Stir in the vegan butter. Adjust salt, lemon juice, or pepper to taste.

Pairs With

Pasta, gnocchi, roasted cherry tomatoes, grilled zucchini, sautéed greens, quinoa bowls, polenta or baked tofu.

Roasted Garlic Alfredo

Creamy, silky, and deeply aromatic, this Alfredo-style sauce blends roasted garlic, cashews, nutmeg, vegan butter, and miso for a rich, savory finish.

Makes About 4 cups | Prep Time 10 minutes | Cook Time 30 minutes

Ingredients

4 heads garlic
8 tablespoons olive oil
2 cups diced onion
4 cups unsweetened plant milk
1½ cups raw cashews*
8 tablespoons nutritional yeast
8 tablespoons lemon juice
2 teaspoons garlic powder
1½ teaspoons fine sea salt
1 teaspoon black pepper
4 tablespoons vegan butter
1 teaspoon nutmeg
4 tablespoons white miso paste
8 cups chopped spinach
8 cups sautéed mushrooms

* soaked in hot water for 10 minutes

Directions

1. Preheat the oven to 400 degrees. Slice the top off each garlic head, drizzle with olive oil, wrap in foil, and roast until soft and golden.
2. Warm the remaining olive oil in a large saucepan and add the diced onion. Cook until softened.
3. Squeeze the roasted garlic cloves into the pan.
4. Add the plant milk, soaked cashews, nutritional yeast, lemon juice, garlic powder, salt, and black pepper.
5. Simmer for 5 minutes.
6. Transfer to a blender and blend until completely smooth.

7. Return the sauce to the saucepan and stir in the vegan butter, nutmeg, miso paste, spinach, and mushrooms.
8. Warm gently and adjust seasoning as needed.

Pairs With

Fettuccine, linguine, gnocchi, roasted broccoli, asparagus, baked tofu, mashed potatoes, lasagna or sautéed greens.

Creamy Sunflower Seed Pasta Sauce

Smooth, neutral, and naturally dairy-free, this nut-free sunflower cream sauce blends roasted peppers, spinach, chili flakes, tahini, and vegan butter for a silky, well-rounded finish that works beautifully with pasta, grains, tofu, or vegetables.

Makes About 4 cups | Prep Time 10 minutes | Cook Time 5 minutes

Ingredients

2 cups raw sunflower seeds*

4 cups unsweetened plant milk

8 cloves garlic

8 tablespoons nutritional yeast

8 tablespoons lemon juice

2 teaspoons onion powder

1 teaspoon black pepper

4 tablespoons vegan butter

4 tablespoons tahini

4 cups roasted red peppers

8 cups fresh spinach

2 teaspoons chili flakes

1½ teaspoons fine sea salt

*soaked in hot water for 10 minutes

Directions

1. Add the soaked sunflower seeds, plant milk, garlic, nutritional yeast, lemon juice, onion powder, salt, and black pepper to a blender.
2. Add the roasted red peppers, spinach, chili flakes, and tahini.
3. Blend until completely smooth and vibrant.
4. Pour the sauce into a saucepan and warm gently over low heat.
5. Stir in the vegan butter until melted and incorporated.
6. Adjust lemon juice, salt, or pepper to taste.

Pairs With

Pasta, gnocchi, roasted vegetables, sautéed greens, quinoa bowls, couscous, tofu cutlets, baked potatoes or grain bowls.

Lemon Tahini Pasta Sauce

Bright, creamy, nutty, and tangy, this lemon-tahini sauce blends garlic, herbs, nutritional yeast, chili flakes, and smoked paprika for a silky, versatile finish that works beautifully with pasta, grains, roasted vegetables, and hearty bowls.

Makes About 4 cups | Prep Time 10 minutes | Cook Time 5 minutes

Ingredients

1½ cups tahini
12 tablespoons lemon juice
1½ cups water
6 garlic cloves, grated
4 tablespoons olive oil
4 tablespoons maple syrup
1½ teaspoons fine sea salt
1 teaspoon black pepper
Zest of 4 lemons
2 teaspoons garlic powder
2 teaspoons chili flakes
8 tablespoons nutritional yeast
1 cup chopped parsley
1 cup chopped basil
2 teaspoons smoked paprika

Directions

1. Add the tahini, lemon juice, water, grated garlic, olive oil, maple syrup, salt, and black pepper to a blender.
2. Add the lemon zest, garlic powder, chili flakes, smoked paprika, nutritional yeast, parsley, and basil. Blend until completely smooth and creamy.
3. Pour the sauce into a saucepan and warm gently over low heat for 2 to 3 minutes, adding more water if needed to reach your preferred consistency.
4. Adjust lemon juice, salt, or pepper to taste.

Pairs With

Pasta, couscous, quinoa, roasted cauliflower, asparagus, broccoli, tofu cutlets, crispy chickpeas, or warm grain bowls.

Mushroom 'Marsala' Pasta Sauce

Rich, savory, and aromatic, this 'Marsala' uses mushrooms, miso, herbs, plant milk, and a touch of balsamic for depth. The sauce stays silky, hearty, and perfect for pasta, tofu, seitan, roasted vegetables, and grain bowls.

Makes About 4 cups | Prep Time 10 minutes | Cook Time 15 minutes

Ingredients

4 tablespoons olive oil

8 cups sliced mushrooms

1½ cups diced onion

8 garlic cloves, minced

2 tablespoons balsamic vinegar

2 tablespoons maple syrup

2 cups unsweetened plant milk

1⅓ cups vegetable broth

4 tablespoons soy sauce or tamari

4 tablespoons nutritional yeast

1½ teaspoons fine sea salt

1 teaspoon black pepper

4 tablespoons vegan butter

4 teaspoons white miso paste

4 teaspoons dried thyme or rosemary

8 cups chopped spinach or kale

2 teaspoons chili flakes

Optional Depth Boosters (Choose 1–2)

1 teaspoon tomato paste

½ teaspoon smoked paprika

½–1 teaspoon cocoa powder (adds depth; blends in)

Directions

1. Warm the olive oil in a large skillet over medium heat.
2. Add the sliced mushrooms and diced onion; cook until browned and softened.
3. Add the minced garlic and cook for 1 minute.
4. Add the balsamic vinegar and maple syrup. Simmer 1–2 minutes to reduce slightly.

5. Add the plant milk, vegetable broth, soy sauce, nutritional yeast, salt, and black pepper.
6. Simmer for 5 to 7 minutes.
7. Stir in the vegan butter until melted.
8. Add the miso paste, dried herbs, spinach or kale, and chili flakes.
9. Warm gently and adjust seasoning to taste.

Pairs With

Pasta, gnocchi, pan-seared tofu, sautéed tempeh, roasted vegetables, mashed potatoes, polenta, farro, or grain bowls.

Caramelized Fennel Pasta Sauce

Subtly sweet, aromatic, and silky, this fennel-flavored sauce blends caramelized fennel, crushed fennel seeds, lemon, greens, roasted tomatoes, and vegan butter into a delicious Mediterranean-inspired sauce..

Makes About 4 cups | Prep Time 10 minutes | Cook Time 20 minutes

Ingredients

4 tablespoons olive oil
4 medium fennel bulbs, thinly sliced
1½ cups diced onion
8 garlic cloves, minced
2 cups vegetable broth
2 cups unsweetened plant milk
4 tablespoons nutritional yeast
4 tablespoons lemon juice
1½ teaspoons fine sea salt
1 teaspoon black pepper
2 teaspoons crushed fennel seeds
4 tablespoons vegan butter
2 teaspoons chili flakes
8 cups fresh peas or spinach
4 cups roasted tomatoes

Directions

1. Warm the olive oil in a large skillet over medium heat. Add the sliced fennel and diced onion and cook until deeply caramelized and golden.
2. Add the garlic and cook for 1 minute. Add the vegetable broth, plant milk, nutritional yeast, lemon juice, fennel seeds, salt, and black pepper.
3. Simmer for 5 minutes. Transfer the mixture to a blender and blend until completely smooth.
4. Return the sauce to the skillet and stir in the vegan butter, chili flakes, peas or spinach, and roasted tomatoes.
5. Warm gently and adjust lemon, salt, or pepper to taste.

Pairs With - Linguine, penne, roasted tomatoes, sautéed greens, tofu cutlets, tempeh, couscous, polenta, or Mediterranean-style grain bowls.

Zesty Roasted Lemon Sauce

Bright, deeply caramelized, and intensely lemony, this sauce blends roasted lemons, garlic, herbs, white beans, chili flakes, and olive oil into a silky, ultra-flavorful finish.

Makes About 4 cups | Prep Time 10 minutes | Cook Time 20 minutes

Ingredients

8 large lemons

8 tablespoons olive oil (for roasting)

16 garlic cloves

1 cup olive oil (for blending)

8 tablespoons lemon juice

4 tablespoons white wine vinegar

1⅓ cups water

1½ teaspoons fine sea salt

1 teaspoon black pepper

2 teaspoons garlic powder

4 tablespoons maple syrup

4 cups cooked white beans

2 cups chopped basil

2 cups chopped parsley

2 teaspoons chili flakes

Directions

1. Preheat the oven to 400 degrees. Slice each lemon into rounds, remove any seeds, lightly coat with olive oil, and roast until soft and caramelized.
2. Add the roasted lemon slices, garlic, olive oil for blending, lemon juice, white wine vinegar, water, salt, and black pepper to a blender.
3. Add the garlic powder, maple syrup, white beans, basil, parsley, and chili flakes. Blend until completely smooth and creamy. Taste and adjust acidity, sweetness, or salt to your liking.

Pairs With

Pasta, roasted asparagus, broccoli, cauliflower, potatoes, quinoa bowls, couscous, tofu cutlets, grilled vegetables or Mediterranean-style salads.

Cashew 'Ricotta' Pasta Sauce

Creamy, mild, and ricotta-inspired, this dairy-free sauce blends cashews, herbs, lemon, roasted garlic, vinegar, and greens into a smooth, versatile finish perfect for pasta, baked shells, lasagna, and vegetable casseroles.

Makes About 4 cups | Prep Time 10 minutes | Cook Time 5 minutes

Ingredients

4 cups raw cashews*

2 cups unsweetened plant milk

8 tablespoons lemon juice

8 tablespoons nutritional yeast

8 garlic cloves

2 teaspoons onion powder

1½ teaspoons fine sea salt

1 teaspoon black pepper

4 tablespoons olive oil

Zest of 2 lemons

4 tablespoons white wine vinegar

8 cups fresh spinach

2 cups chopped basil

2 cups chopped parsley

8 tablespoons roasted garlic

* soaked in hot water for 10 minutes

Directions

1. Add the soaked cashews, plant milk, lemon juice, nutritional yeast, garlic cloves, onion powder, salt, and black pepper to a blender.
2. Add the olive oil, lemon zest, white wine vinegar, spinach, basil, parsley, and roasted garlic.
3. Blend until completely smooth and creamy.
4. Pour the sauce into a saucepan and warm gently over low heat for 3 to 5 minutes. Adjust lemon, salt, or pepper as needed.

Pairs With

Pasta, baked shells, lasagna layers, stuffed vegetables, gnocchi, roasted zucchini, eggplant, tofu cutlets or polenta bowls.

Creamy Garlic Herb Mushroom Sauce

This rich, velvety creation transforms garlic, herbs, mushrooms, and capers into a creamy white sauce.

Makes About 4 cups | Prep Time 10 minutes | Cook Time 10 minutes

Ingredients

4 tablespoons olive oil

12 garlic cloves, minced

8 cups sliced mushrooms

1½ cups vegetable broth

1 cup unsweetened plant milk (cashew, oat, or soy work best)

½ cup plain, unsweetened dairy-free yogurt *or* ½ cup cashew cream

4 tablespoons lemon juice

3 tablespoons vegan butter

1½ teaspoons fine sea salt

1 teaspoon black pepper

2 teaspoons dried thyme

2 teaspoons dried oregano

2 teaspoons chili flakes

1 cup capers

1 cup chopped fresh parsley

Optional Cream-Boosting Add-Ins

2–3 tablespoons nutritional yeast

2 tablespoons cashew butter or tahini

1 teaspoon white miso (for extra savoriness)

½ teaspoon mustard powder

Directions

1. Warm the olive oil in a large skillet over medium heat.
2. Add the garlic and cook until fragrant.
3. Add the mushrooms and cook until softened and lightly browned.
4. Add the vegetable broth, plant milk, lemon juice, thyme, oregano, salt, and pepper.
5. Simmer 3–4 minutes, allowing the mixture to thicken slightly.
6. Reduce heat to low and stir in the vegan butter and dairy-free yogurt (or cashew cream).
7. Add the capers, chili flakes, and parsley.
8. Warm gently until the sauce becomes silky.
9. Stir in any optional cream-boosting add-ins and adjust seasoning to taste.

Pairs With

Creamy linguine, gnocchi, roasted asparagus, tofu cutlets, sautéed greens, white beans, couscous, or vegetable medleys.

Bruschetta Pasta Sauce

Fresh, bright, and full of tomato flavor, this warm bruschetta-inspired sauce blends fresh tomatoes, balsamic vinegar, basil, olives, chili flakes, vegan butter, and roasted cherry tomatoes for a bold, savory finish perfect for pasta and roasted vegetables.

Makes About 4 cups | Prep Time 10 minutes | Cook Time 10 minutes

Ingredients

4 tablespoons olive oil

12 garlic cloves, minced

16 cups chopped tomatoes, diced

2 cups fresh basil, chopped

8 tablespoons balsamic vinegar

4 tablespoons olive oil (for finishing)

4 teaspoons garlic powder

2 teaspoons onion powder

1½ teaspoons fine sea salt

1 teaspoon black pepper

4 tablespoons vegan butter

2 teaspoons chili flakes

8 cups roasted cherry tomatoes

4 cups sliced olives

4 cups cooked white beans

Directions

1. Warm the olive oil in a large saucepan over medium heat. Add the minced garlic and cook until fragrant.
2. Add the chopped tomatoes, garlic powder, onion powder, salt, and black pepper. Simmer for 8 to 10 minutes, stirring occasionally.
3. Stir in the balsamic vinegar, fresh basil, vegan butter, chili flakes, roasted cherry tomatoes, olives, and white beans.
4. Warm gently until everything is combined and heated through. Adjust salt, pepper, or balsamic to taste.

Pairs With - Pasta, gnocchi, roasted zucchini, eggplant, white beans, bruschetta bowls, polenta or Mediterranean-style grain bowls.

4. Curry Sauces

Curry sauces bring warmth, depth, and aromatic richness to plant-based cooking, transforming even simple ingredients into satisfying meals. Whether coconut or tomato based, herb-filled or layered with aromatic spices, these versatile sauces meet a wide range of tastes and flavors.

Spoon them over rice, quinoa, noodles, roasted vegetables, tofu, tempeh, chickpeas, or sautéed greens, or use them as simmer sauces for quick weeknight curries. Each recipe in this section delivers bold flavor in a small batch, perfect for adding a vibrant finishing touch to any vegan dish.

- Thai Red Curry Sauce
- Golden Curry Cashew Sauce
- Tomato Coconut Curry Sauce
- Green Herb Coconut Curry Sauce
- Sweet Potato Curry Sauce

Thai Red Curry Coconut Sauce

Silky, aromatic, and restaurant-style — perfect for noodles, rice bowls, tofu, vegetables, and simmered curries.

Makes About 2 cups | Prep Time 10 minutes | Cook Time 10 minutes

Ingredients

1 tablespoon coconut oil

2 tablespoons red curry paste

2 cloves garlic, minced

1 teaspoon grated fresh ginger

1 can (13.5 ounces) full-fat coconut milk

1 tablespoon soy sauce or tamari

1 tablespoon lime juice

1 teaspoon maple syrup

1 teaspoon turmeric

½ teaspoon salt

¼ teaspoon black pepper

1 tablespoon chopped fresh cilantro (optional garnish)

Directions

1. Warm coconut oil in a saucepan over medium heat.
2. Stir in red curry paste, garlic, and ginger; cook 1 minute.
3. Add coconut milk, soy sauce, lime juice, maple syrup, turmeric, salt, and black pepper.
4. Simmer 5 minutes, stirring. Taste and adjust lime or salt.

Golden Curry Cashew Sauce

Creamy, bright, and lightly spiced — perfect over rice, chickpeas, vegetables, or noodles.

Makes About About 2 cups | Prep Time 10 minutes | Cook Time 5 minutes

Ingredients

1 tablespoon olive oil

½ cup diced onion

2 cloves garlic, minced

1 teaspoon grated ginger

1 tablespoon curry powder

½ teaspoon turmeric

½ cup raw cashews, soaked 10 minutes

1½ cups unsweetened plant milk

1 tablespoon lemon juice

½ teaspoon salt

¼ teaspoon black pepper

Directions

1. Warm olive oil in a saucepan and add the onion. Cook until softened.
2. Add garlic, ginger, curry powder, and turmeric; cook 1 minute.
3. Add plant milk, cashews, lemon juice, salt, and pepper.
4. Simmer 3 to 5 minutes.
5. Blend until smooth.

Tomato Coconut Curry Sauce

A rich, restaurant-style tomato curry blending coconut milk, aromatics, and warm spices.

Makes About 2 cups | Prep Time 10 minutes | Cook Time 12 minutes

Ingredients

1 tablespoon olive oil

½ cup diced onion

2 cloves garlic, minced

1 teaspoon grated ginger

1 teaspoon garam masala

1 teaspoon curry powder

½ teaspoon cumin

1 cup crushed tomatoes

1 cup coconut milk

½ teaspoon salt

¼ teaspoon pepper

1 teaspoon maple syrup

Directions

1. Warm olive oil in a saucepan and cook the onion until soft.
2. Add garlic and ginger; cook 1 minute.
3. Stir in garam masala, curry powder, and cumin.
4. Add crushed tomatoes, coconut milk, salt, pepper, and maple syrup.
5. Simmer 8 minutes.

Green Herb Coconut Curry Sauce

Fresh, herbal and vibrant — great for vegetables, tofu, noodles, or grain bowls.

Makes About 2 cups | Prep Time 10 minutes | Cook Time 5 minutes

Ingredients

1 can (13.5 ounces) coconut milk

1 cup fresh spinach

½ cup fresh cilantro

¼ cup fresh basil

2 green onions, chopped

1 tablespoon lime juice

1 tablespoon soy sauce or tamari

1 teaspoon grated ginger

2 cloves garlic

1 teaspoon curry powder

¼ teaspoon salt

Chili flakes to taste

Directions

1. Add all ingredients to a blender and blend until smooth.
2. Pour into a saucepan and warm 3 to 5 minutes.
3. Adjust lime or salt.

Sweet Potato Curry Sauce

Creamy, hearty, and naturally sweet — perfect for fall bowls, chickpeas, tofu, or roasted vegetables.

Makes About 2 cups | Prep Time 10 minutes | Cook Time 12 minutes

Ingredients

1 tablespoon olive oil

½ cup diced onion

2 cloves garlic, minced

1 teaspoon grated ginger

1 cup mashed cooked sweet potato

1 tablespoon curry powder

½ teaspoon smoked paprika

1 cup vegetable broth

½ cup coconut milk

½ teaspoon salt

¼ teaspoon pepper

1 teaspoon maple syrup

Directions

1. Warm olive oil in a saucepan and cook the onion until soft.
2. Add garlic and ginger.
3. Stir in sweet potato, curry powder, smoked paprika, broth, coconut milk, salt, and pepper.
4. Simmer for 8 minutes. Blend for a smoother finish.

5. Tofu-Based and Protein-Boosted Sauces

Smooth, high-protein sauces that bring body and nourishment without nuts — ideal for pasta, drizzles, or creamy bowl toppings.

Smooth, high-protein, and adaptable — tofu makes a perfect base for creamy, dairy-free sauces. It blends effortlessly into alfredos, aiolis, and smoky drizzles that can be used warm or cold. These recipes prove that protein and creaminess can live side-by-side, naturally.

- Silken Tofu Alfredo
- Tofu Garlic Lemon Sauce
- Spicy Tofu Aioli
- Creamy Basil Tofu Sauce
- Smoky Tofu Cream

Silken Tofu Alfredo

Creamy, garlicky, and light — this dairy-free take on Alfredo sauce coats pasta beautifully and reheats well without separating.

Makes About 2 cups | Prep Time 10 minutes | Cook Time 10 minutes

Ingredients

1 package (12 ounces) silken tofu, drained

2 tablespoons olive oil

2 cloves garlic, minced

2 tablespoons nutritional yeast

2 tablespoons lemon juice

1 teaspoon Dijon mustard

½ teaspoon salt

¼ teaspoon black pepper

¼ cup unsweetened plant milk

Directions

1. Heat olive oil in a skillet over medium heat. Add garlic and cook 1 minute until fragrant.
2. Transfer to a blender with tofu, nutritional yeast, lemon juice, mustard, salt, pepper and plant milk. Blend until completely smooth.
3. Return to pan and warm over low heat 3–5 minutes. Stir until thickened.

Make It Yours Ideas

Add a tablespoon of vegan butter for richness or a pinch of nutmeg for depth. Add crushed red pepper for a mild kick.

Pairs With

Fettuccine, sautéed mushrooms, roasted asparagus, or steamed broccoli.

Tofu Garlic Lemon Sauce

Bright, tangy, and smooth, this sauce complements roasted vegetables and bowls while adding a gentle protein boost.

Makes About 2 cups | Prep Time 10 minutes | Cook Time 5 minutes

Ingredients

1 package (14 ounces) firm tofu, drained

¼ cup olive oil

Juice of 1 large lemon (about 3 tablespoons)

2 cloves garlic

1 teaspoon maple syrup

½ teaspoon salt

¼ teaspoon black pepper

¼ cup warm water

Directions

Blend tofu, olive oil, lemon juice, garlic, maple syrup, salt, pepper, and water until smooth and creamy. Warm gently in a saucepan for 3–5 minutes, stirring constantly until thickened.

Make It Yours Ideas

Add 2 tablespoons nutritional yeast for a richer flavor. Blend in a pinch of cayenne or a spoonful of prepared horseradish.

Pairs With

Roasted vegetables, grain bowls, grilled tempeh, or vegan crab cakes.

Spicy Tofu Aioli

A bold and tangy sauce that gives burgers, fries, and sandwiches a creamy, kicky finish — no mayo required.

Makes About 2 cups | Prep Time 10 minutes | Cook Time 5 minutes

Ingredients

1 package (12 ounces) silken tofu, drained

2 tablespoons olive oil

1 tablespoon lemon juice

1 tablespoon apple cider vinegar

1 tablespoon sriracha or chili-garlic sauce

1 garlic clove

½ teaspoon salt

¼ teaspoon smoked paprika

Directions

Blend tofu, olive oil, lemon juice, vinegar, sriracha, garlic, salt, and smoked paprika until smooth. Warm gently in a small saucepan over low heat for 3–4 minutes, stirring occasionally, until creamy and slightly thickened.

Make It Yours Ideas

Add 1 tablespoon Dijon mustard or extra lemon juice for a tangier version. Double the sriracha or use chipotle paste for a smoky twist.

Pairs With

Veggie burgers, fries, roasted cauliflower, or wraps.

Creamy Basil Tofu Sauce

Fresh basil transforms simple tofu into a luscious, herb-packed sauce reminiscent of pesto but lighter and higher in protein.

Makes About 2 cups | Prep Time 10 minutes | Cook Time 5 minutes

Ingredients

1 package (12 ounces) silken tofu, drained

1 cup fresh basil leaves, loosely packed

2 tablespoons olive oil

1 tablespoon lemon juice

1 garlic clove

2 tablespoons nutritional yeast

½ teaspoon salt

¼ teaspoon black pepper

Directions

Blend tofu, basil, olive oil, lemon juice, garlic, nutritional yeast, salt, and pepper until smooth and bright green. Warm gently in a small saucepan 3–5 minutes over low heat, stirring to thicken slightly.

Make It Yours Ideas

Substitute half the basil with baby spinach for a milder flavor. Add red pepper flakes or a touch of jalapeño.

Pairs With

Pasta, grain bowls, roasted tomatoes, or vegan mozzarella.

Smoky Tofu Cream

This deeply savory sauce delivers richness with just the right touch of smoke — a versatile base for barbecue bowls, baked potatoes, or grilled vegetables.

Makes About 2 cups | Prep Time 10 minutes | Cook Time 10 minutes

Ingredients

1 package (14 ounces) firm tofu, drained

2 tablespoons olive oil

1 tablespoon lemon juice

1 tablespoon tomato paste

1 teaspoon smoked paprika

½ teaspoon garlic powder

½ teaspoon onion powder

¼ teaspoon liquid smoke (or more to taste)

½ teaspoon salt

¼ teaspoon black pepper

¼ cup warm water

Directions

Blend tofu, olive oil, lemon juice, tomato paste, smoked paprika, garlic powder, onion powder, liquid smoke, salt, pepper, and water until smooth. Transfer to a small saucepan and heat 5–7 minutes, stirring until creamy and slightly thickened.

Make It Yours Ideas

Add 1 tablespoon maple syrup for a sweet-smoky barbecue note. Blend in chili powder or cayenne for extra warmth.

Pairs With

BBQ cauliflower wings, roasted sweet potatoes, or lentil patties.

6. Nut and Seed-Based Sauces

Creamy, nutrient-rich blends that bring depth, body, and a natural balance of protein and flavor to your vegan kitchen.

Bold and flavorful, these sauces turn humble nuts and seeds into the backbone of your flavor palette. From a rich peanut satay to smoky walnut spreads, each recipe offers plant-based protein, healthy fats, and deep, craveable flavor — all made with simple pantry ingredients.

- Peanut Satay Sauce
- Almond Ginger Sauce
- Sunflower Seed Dressing
- Sesame Miso Sauce
- Walnut and Roasted Garlic Spread

Peanut Satay Sauce

A smooth, savory-sweet sauce that's delicious over noodles, tofu, or roasted vegetables — inspired by Southeast Asian street flavors but simplified for everyday cooking.

Makes About 2 cups | Prep Time 10 minutes | Cook Time 10 minutes

Ingredients

¾ cup natural peanut butter (unsweetened, smooth or chunky)

1 cup warm water, plus more to thin

2 tablespoons low-sodium soy sauce or tamari

1 tablespoon maple syrup or agave

1 tablespoon lime juice

1 clove garlic, minced

1 teaspoon grated fresh ginger

½ teaspoon chili flakes or 1 teaspoon sriracha (optional)

Directions

1. Whisk all ingredients in a small saucepan over medium heat until smooth and gently bubbling, 5–7 minutes.
2. Add a splash of water to thin as desired. Remove from heat and cool slightly before serving.

Make It Yours Ideas

Replace peanut butter with almond butter or sunflower seed butter. Add extra chili flakes or a chili-garlic paste for a bolder version.

Pairs With

Rice noodles, tofu skewers, roasted sweet potatoes, or Buddha bowls.

Almond Ginger Sauce

Light and aromatic with notes of ginger, garlic, and citrus — this sauce adds elegance to stir-fries and roasted vegetables.

Makes About 2 cups | Prep Time 10 minutes | Cook Time 5 minutes

Ingredients

¾ cup raw almonds (soaked 2 hours or blanched)

¾ cup warm water

1 tablespoon sesame oil

1 tablespoon tamari or soy sauce

1 tablespoon lime juice

1 teaspoon grated fresh ginger

1 garlic clove

1 tablespoon maple syrup

1 teaspoon rice vinegar

Pinch of red pepper flakes

Directions

Blend soaked almonds, warm water, sesame oil, tamari, lime juice, ginger, garlic, maple syrup, vinegar, and red pepper flakes until smooth and creamy. Warm gently in a small pan 3–4 minutes to combine flavors.

Make It Yours Ideas

Add 1 tablespoon of toasted sesame seeds or 1 teaspoon miso paste for richness. Stir in extra ginger or a few drops of chili oil.

Pairs With

Stir-fried greens, soba noodles, steamed dumplings, or grilled tofu.

Sunflower Seed Dressing

A creamy, nut-free alternative with a mellow, earthy flavor that pairs beautifully with bowls and wraps.

Makes About 2 cups | Prep Time 10 minutes | Cook Time 5 minutes

Ingredients

¾ cup raw sunflower seeds (soaked 2 hours)

¾ cup warm water

1 garlic clove

2 tablespoons lemon juice

1 tablespoon apple cider vinegar

2 teaspoons Dijon mustard

½ teaspoon salt

¼ teaspoon black pepper

2 tablespoons olive oil

Directions

Blend soaked sunflower seeds, warm water, garlic, lemon juice, vinegar, mustard, salt, pepper, and olive oil until creamy and smooth. Warm gently on low heat 3–5 minutes to bring flavors together.

Make It Yours Ideas

Add a handful of fresh herbs like parsley or cilantro for a green version.

Stir in ½ teaspoon smoked paprika or chili powder.

Pairs With

Roasted vegetables, quinoa bowls, or lentil patties.

Sesame Miso Sauce

A rich and umami-packed sauce with deep sesame flavor, balanced by salty-sweet miso and maple.

Makes About 2 cups | Prep Time 10 minutes | Cook Time 5 minutes

Ingredients

¼ cup tahini

2 tablespoons white or yellow miso paste

1 tablespoon rice vinegar

1 tablespoon soy sauce or tamari

1 tablespoon maple syrup

1 teaspoon toasted sesame oil

¾ cup warm water

1 clove garlic, minced

½ teaspoon grated ginger

Directions

Whisk all ingredients in a small saucepan over medium-low heat until smooth and warmed through, about 5 minutes. Add more water for a thinner consistency if desired.

Make It Yours Ideas

Add 1 tablespoon lime juice or a spoonful of peanut butter for a Southeast Asian twist.

Stir in chili oil or shichimi togarashi (a 7-ingredient Japanese spice blend) for heat.

Pairs With

Grain bowls, grilled vegetables, tofu, or cold noodle salads.

Walnut and Roasted Garlic Spread

Hearty, savory, and deeply aromatic — this spread doubles as a sauce for pasta or a flavorful layer for sandwiches.

Makes About 2 cups | Prep Time 10 minutes | Cook Time 25 minutes

Ingredients

1 cup walnuts

1 small head garlic

2 tablespoons olive oil, divided

2 tablespoons lemon juice

½ teaspoon salt and ¼ teaspoon black pepper

½ cup warm water

1 tablespoon tomato paste (optional for color and balance)

Directions

1. Preheat oven to 400°F. Slice off the top of the garlic head to expose cloves, drizzle with 1 tablespoon olive oil and wrap in foil. Roast 20–25 minutes until soft.
2. Toast walnuts on a baking sheet for 5–7 minutes until fragrant. Blend roasted garlic (skins removed) with walnuts, remaining olive oil, lemon juice, salt, pepper, water, and tomato paste until smooth but textured.
3. Warm gently in a saucepan 3–5 minutes to meld flavors.

Make It Yours Ideas

Add fresh parsley or basil before blending. Stir in a pinch of chili flakes or smoked paprika.

Pairs With

Pasta, roasted vegetables, or as a sandwich spread.

7. Comfort Sauces and Gravies

Comfort sauces and gravies bring warmth, richness, and depth to simple meals — the kind of flavors that make a dish feel complete.

These sauces cover vegetables, mushrooms, potatoes, and bowls with familiar, satisfying notes of savory herbs, caramelized onions, and slow-simmered goodness. Whether you're pouring a silky gravy over portabella "steaks," stirring a creamy sauce into mashed potatoes, or adding a spoonful to roasted vegetables, these recipes turn everyday plantsy ingredients into homey, nourishing comfort food.

- Homemade Cranberry Sauce
- Slow Cooker Cranberry Sauce
- Savory Cranberry Herb Gravy
- Salisbury Style Slow Cooker Gravy
- Slow Cooker Savory Mushroom Gravy
- Cashew Cream Comfort Gravy
- Tofu Cream Country Gravy
- Mediterranean Herb Gravy
- Caramelized Onion Gravy
- Peppercorn Gravy
- Miso Rosemary Gravy
- Smoky Paprika Gravy
- Garlic Sage Gravy
- Herb Tahini Gravy
- Creamy Garlic Gravy
- Onion Miso Gravy
- Coconut Pepper Gravy
- Rosemary Shallot Gravy

Homemade Cranberry Sauce

Bright, tart, and gently sweet — a simple sauce that brings balance to savory dishes and adds sparkle to holiday or everyday meals.

Makes About 2 cups | Prep Time 5 minutes | Cook Time 12–15 minutes

Ingredients

2 cups fresh cranberries (or frozen)

½ cup water

½ cup maple syrup or coconut sugar

1 tablespoon orange juice

1 teaspoon orange zest

¼ teaspoon cinnamon

Pinch of salt

Directions

Combine cranberries, water, maple syrup, orange juice, orange zest, cinnamon, and salt in a saucepan. Bring to a simmer over medium heat. Cook 12–15 minutes, stirring occasionally, until cranberries burst and the sauce thickens. Cool before serving.

Slow Cooker Cranberry Sauce

A hands-off version that develops deeper flavor and a jammy texture — perfect for meal prep, holiday cooking, or convenience.

Makes About 2 cups | Prep Time 5 minutes | Cook Time 3 hours

Ingredients

2 cups fresh or frozen cranberries

½ cup water

½ cup maple syrup or coconut sugar

1 tablespoon orange juice

1 teaspoon orange zest

¼ teaspoon cinnamon

Pinch of salt

Directions

Add cranberries, water, maple syrup, orange juice, orange zest, cinnamon, and salt to a slow cooker. Stir, cover, and cook on Low for 3 hours, stirring once halfway through. Cool before serving.

Make It Yours Ideas

Stir in chopped apples during the last hour for a thicker, chunkier texture or add 1–2 tablespoons chopped walnuts after cooling.

Add ground ginger, nutmeg, cardamom or a pinch of cloves.

Pairs With

Portabella or cauliflower steaks, holiday plates, roasted vegetables, grain bowls, mashed potatoes, yogurt, or toast.

Savory Cranberry Herb Gravy

A bright, tangy, savory twist on classic gravy, it balances richness with a pop of cranberry and herbs.

Makes About 2 cups | Prep Time 10 minutes | Cook Time 12 minutes

Ingredients

1 tablespoon olive oil or vegan butter

½ cup finely diced onion

2 cloves garlic, minced

2 tablespoons flour

1 ½ cups vegetable broth

⅓ cup whole cranberry sauce (homemade or store-bought)

1 tablespoon soy sauce or coconut aminos

1 teaspoon dried thyme

½ teaspoon dried sage

½ teaspoon dried rosemary

½ teaspoon salt and ¼ teaspoon black pepper

Directions

Warm olive oil in a saucepan. Add onion and sauté 5 minutes. Add garlic and cook 1 minute. Stir in flour to form a paste. Slowly whisk in vegetable broth.

Add cranberry sauce, soy sauce, thyme, sage, rosemary, salt, and pepper. Simmer 8–10 minutes until thick and glossy.

Make It Yours Ideas

Use fresh herbs instead of dried for a more aromatic finish. Add a pinch of cayenne or smoked paprika for a deeper flavor.

Pairs With

Portabella steaks, mashed potatoes, roasted carrots or lentil loaves.

Salisbury Style Slow Cooker Gravy

A comforting, savory plant-based entrée with deep flavor and a tenderness.

Serves: 4 large mushrooms | Prep Time 10 minutes | Cook Time Slow Cooker 2–3 hours OR Oven 40 minutes

Ingredients

4 extra large portabella mushrooms, stems removed

1 tablespoon olive oil

½ teaspoon salt

½ teaspoon black pepper

½ teaspoon garlic powder

½ teaspoon onion powder

1 full batch of *Savory Mushroom Gravy* (recipe below)

Directions

Brush mushrooms with olive oil and sprinkle with salt, pepper, garlic powder, and onion powder. Place mushrooms gill-side up in a slow cooker or baking dish. Pour the gravy over the mushrooms.

If slow cooking: cook on Low for 2–3 hours.
If baking: cover dish and bake at 325°F for 40 minutes.

Serve warm with mashed potatoes, roasted vegetables, or rice.

Make It Yours Ideas

Add sliced onions and mushrooms to the slow cooker for a chunky, stew-like finish. Add a pinch of smoked paprika.

Pairs With

Mashed potatoes, green beans, roasted carrots, or biscuits.

Slow Cooker Savory Mushroom Gravy

Rich, hearty, deeply savory — this gravy captures the flavor of classic Salisbury Steak gravies using clean, homemade ingredients. It's designed to cling beautifully to large portabella mushrooms, tofu steaks, lentil patties, or mashed potatoes.

Makes About 2 cups | Prep Time 10 minutes | Cook Time 15 minutes (or longer if simmering with portabellas)

Ingredients

2 tablespoons vegan butter or olive oil

½ cup finely diced onion

½ cup sliced mushrooms (baby bella or cremini)

2 cloves garlic, minced

2 tablespoons flour (all-purpose or whole wheat)

1 ½ cups vegetable broth

1 tablespoon soy sauce or coconut aminos

1 teaspoon Dijon mustard

1 teaspoon dried onion flakes

1 teaspoon dried parsley

½ teaspoon dried thyme

½ teaspoon paprika

¼ teaspoon black pepper

¼ teaspoon smoked paprika (optional)

¼ cup unsweetened plant milk OR 2 tablespoons cashew cream (for richness)

Directions

1. Warm vegan butter in a saucepan. Add onion and mushrooms and sauté 5–7 minutes until soft and golden. Add garlic and cook 1 minute. Sprinkle in flour and stir to coat, forming a paste.

2. Add vegetable broth slowly while whisking. Stir in soy sauce, mustard, dried onion flakes, parsley, thyme, paprika, pepper, and smoked paprika. Simmer 8–10 minutes, stirring often, until thick and glossy.
3. Stir in plant milk or cashew cream for richness.
4. Taste and adjust seasoning.

Make It Yours Ideas

Add ½ teaspoon of vegan Worcestershire-style sauce or a splash of balsamic for extra depth.

Add a pinch of cayenne or crushed black pepper for heat.

Pairs With

Portabella mushrooms, mashed potatoes, lentil loaves, tofu steaks, roasted root vegetables.

Cashew Cream Comfort Gravy

Thick, rich, and ultra-smooth.

Makes About 2 cups | Prep Time 10 minutes | Cook Time 10 minutes

Ingredients

1 tablespoon olive oil

½ cup finely chopped onion

2 cloves garlic

2 tablespoons flour

1 ½ cups vegetable broth

¼ cup cashews, soaked 20 minutes

1 tablespoon soy sauce or coconut aminos

½ teaspoon thyme

½ teaspoon paprika

½ teaspoon salt

Directions

Sauté onion and garlic in olive oil 4–5 minutes. Add flour and cook 1 minute. Pour broth in slowly. Blend soaked cashews with ¼ cup hot broth until smooth. Add to pot. Simmer until thick and glossy.

Pairs With

Portabella steaks, mashed potatoes or biscuits.

Tofu Cream Country Gravy

Light, creamy, and perfect for smothering.

Makes About 2 cups | Prep Time 10 minutes

Ingredients

½ cup soft tofu

1 ½ cups vegetable broth

2 tablespoons nutritional yeast

2 tablespoons flour

1 tablespoon soy sauce

1 teaspoon garlic powder

1 teaspoon onion powder

½ teaspoon thyme

½ teaspoon salt

Directions

Blend tofu until smooth. Whisk with broth, nutritional yeast, flour, soy sauce, garlic powder, onion powder, thyme, and salt in a saucepan. Simmer 8–10 minutes until thickened.

Pairs With

Portabella steaks, biscuits, rice bowls.

Mediterranean Herb Gravy

A bright, aromatic variation with Mediterranean flair.

Makes About 2 cups | Prep Time 10 minutes | Cook Time 10 minutes

Ingredients

1 tablespoon olive oil

½ cup finely chopped onion

2 cloves garlic

2 tablespoons flour

1 ½ cups vegetable broth

1 tablespoon lemon juice

1 tablespoon chopped parsley

1 teaspoon oregano

1 teaspoon basil

½ teaspoon thyme

½ teaspoon salt

¼ teaspoon black pepper

Directions

Sauté onion and garlic in olive oil 4 minutes. Add flour and cook 1 minute. Slowly whisk in broth. Add lemon juice, parsley, oregano, basil, thyme, salt, and pepper. Simmer 8–10 minutes until thickened.

Pairs With

Portabella steaks, roasted potatoes, chickpeas, Mediterranean bowls.

Caramelized Onion Gravy

Sweet, savory, and full of depth — this gravy gets its body and richness from slowly cooked onions.

Makes About 2 cups | Prep Time 10 minutes | Cook Time 20 minutes

Ingredients

1 tablespoon olive oil or vegan butter

2 large onions, thinly sliced

2 cloves garlic, minced

2 tablespoons flour

1 ½ cups vegetable broth

1 tablespoon soy sauce or coconut aminos

½ teaspoon dried thyme

½ teaspoon salt and ¼ teaspoon black pepper

Directions

1. Warm olive oil in a saucepan. Add onions and cook 12–15 minutes, stirring often, until deeply golden. Add garlic and cook 1 minute. Sprinkle in flour and stir to coat.
2. Slowly pour in broth while whisking. Add soy sauce, thyme, salt, and pepper. Simmer 5–7 minutes until thick and glossy.

Make It Yours Ideas

Blend half or all of the gravy for a smoother texture.

Add smoked paprika or a splash of balsamic vinegar.

Pairs With

Mashed potatoes, roasted vegetables, savory loaves, and biscuits.

Peppercorn Gravy

Bold, creamy, and deeply savory — inspired by classic steakhouse peppercorn sauce, but made 100% plantsy.

Makes About 2 cups | Prep Time 10 minutes | Cook Time 10 minutes

Ingredients

1 tablespoon vegan butter or olive oil

½ cup finely diced onion

2 cloves garlic, minced

2 tablespoons flour

1 ½ cups vegetable broth

¼ cup unsweetened plant milk or 2 tablespoons cashew cream

1 tablespoon soy sauce

1 tablespoon crushed black peppercorns (coarse-cracked)

½ teaspoon salt

Directions

Warm butter in a saucepan. Add onion and sauté 5 minutes. Add garlic and cook 1 minute. Stir in flour to form a paste. Whisk in vegetable broth. Add plant milk, soy sauce, peppercorns and salt. Simmer 8–10 minutes until thickened.

Make It Yours Ideas

Blend half the gravy to make it even smoother, then stir back in.

Add a pinch of cayenne or smoked pepper.

Pairs With

Portabella steaks, mashed potatoes, tofu steaks, and roasted cauliflower.

Miso Rosemary Gravy

Rich, earthy, and aromatic — combining the umami of miso with the herbal warmth of rosemary. A perfect match for mushrooms.

Makes About 2 cups | Prep Time 10 minutes | Cook Time 10 minutes

Ingredients

1 tablespoon olive oil

½ cup finely chopped onion

2 cloves garlic, minced

2 tablespoons flour

1 ½ cups vegetable broth

1 tablespoon white miso

1 tablespoon soy sauce or coconut aminos

1 teaspoon chopped fresh rosemary

½ teaspoon dried thyme

½ teaspoon salt

¼ teaspoon black pepper

Directions

Warm olive oil in a saucepan. Add onion and sauté 5 minutes. Add garlic and cook 1 minute. Stir in flour. Pour in vegetable broth slowly while whisking. Add miso, soy sauce, rosemary, thyme, salt, and pepper. Simmer 8–10 minutes until creamy and fragrant.

Make It Yours Ideas

Swap rosemary for sage or oregano for a different herbal profile. Add a pinch of crushed red pepper or smoked paprika.

Pairs With

Portabella steaks, roasted potatoes, root vegetables, chickpea cutlets.

Smoky Paprika Gravy

Deep, warm, and full of smoky flavor.

Makes About 2 cups | Prep Time 10 minutes | Cook Time 10 minutes

Ingredients

1 tablespoon olive oil or vegan butter

½ cup finely diced onion

2 cloves garlic, minced

2 tablespoons flour

1 ½ cups vegetable broth

2 tablespoons tomato paste

1 teaspoon smoked paprika

½ teaspoon regular paprika

1 tablespoon soy sauce or coconut aminos

½ teaspoon salt

¼ teaspoon black pepper

Directions

Warm olive oil in a saucepan. Add onion and cook 5 minutes. Add garlic and cook 1 minute. Sprinkle in flour and stir to form a paste. Whisk in vegetable broth slowly. Add tomato paste, smoked paprika, paprika, soy sauce, salt, and pepper. Simmer 8–10 minutes until thickened and smoky.

Make It Yours Ideas

Stir in a tablespoon of cashew cream for extra richness.

Add chipotle powder or a pinch of cayenne.

Pairs With - Portabella steaks, hearty bowls, grilled or roasted vegetables, roasted potatoes, chickpeas, or couscous.

Garlic Sage Gravy

A warm, aromatic gravy that works well with roasted vegetables, mashed potatoes, mushroom steaks, and tofu.

Makes about 1 cup | Prep Time 5 minutes | Cook Time 10 minutes

Ingredients

1 tablespoon olive oil

3 cloves garlic, minced

1 tablespoon all-purpose flour

1 cup vegetable broth

1 teaspoon dried sage or 1 tablespoon finely chopped fresh sage

½ teaspoon onion powder

Black pepper to taste

Salt if needed

Directions

1. Heat the olive oil in a small saucepan over medium heat.
2. Add the garlic and cook 1 minute.
3. Add the flour and whisk to form a paste.
4. Pour in the vegetable broth while whisking.
5. Add the sage and onion powder.
6. Cook 6–8 minutes until thickened.
7. Taste and adjust seasoning.

Herb Tahini Gravy

Creamy, nutty, and herby — a Mediterranean-inspired gravy perfect for bowls, roasted vegetables, and potatoes.

Makes About 2 cups | Prep Time 5 minutes | Cook Time 5 minutes

Ingredients

½ cup tahini

1 ½ cups vegetable broth

2 tablespoons lemon juice

1 tablespoon soy sauce or coconut aminos

1 tablespoon chopped fresh parsley

1 teaspoon dried oregano

½ teaspoon garlic powder

½ teaspoon salt and ¼ teaspoon black pepper

Directions

Whisk tahini and vegetable broth in a saucepan over medium heat until smooth. Add lemon juice, soy sauce, parsley, oregano, garlic powder, salt, and pepper. Cook 3–5 minutes until warmed and slightly thickened.

Make It Yours Ideas

Use fresh oregano or dill for a brighter, fresher flavor.

Add Aleppo pepper or smoked paprika.

Pairs With

Roasted vegetables, grain bowls, potatoes, tofu steaks, or warm pita.

Creamy Garlic Gravy

Smooth, mellow, and full of roasted-garlic flavor — a classic comfort gravy in fully plant-based form.

Makes About 2 cups | Prep Time 10 minutes | Cook Time 15 minutes

Ingredients

1 tablespoon vegan butter or olive oil

1 head garlic, roasted

2 tablespoons flour

1 ½ cups vegetable broth

½ cup unsweetened plant milk or 2 tablespoons cashew cream

1 tablespoon nutritional yeast

½ teaspoon salt

¼ teaspoon black pepper

Directions

Squeeze roasted garlic from the skins. Warm butter in a saucepan. Add roasted garlic and mash lightly with a spoon. Add flour and stir to form a paste. Slowly whisk in vegetable broth. Add plant milk, nutritional yeast, salt, and pepper. Simmer 10–12 minutes until thick and creamy.

Make It Yours Ideas

Blend the gravy for an ultra-smooth finish.

Add a pinch of nutmeg or smoked paprika.

Pairs With

Mashed potatoes, roasted vegetables, biscuits, mushrooms, tofu steaks.

Onion Miso Gravy

Savory, rich, and umami-packed — this gravy brings deep flavor without heaviness. It pairs nicely with mushrooms, roasted vegetables, and grain bowls.

Makes About 2 cups | Prep Time 10 minutes | Cook Time 15 minutes

Ingredients

1 tablespoon olive oil or vegan butter

1 large onion, thinly sliced

2 cloves garlic, minced

2 tablespoons flour

1 ½ cups vegetable broth

1 tablespoon white miso

1 tablespoon soy sauce or coconut aminos

½ teaspoon dried thyme

½ teaspoon salt

¼ teaspoon black pepper

Directions

Warm oil in a saucepan. Add sliced onion and cook 10–12 minutes, stirring often, until deeply golden. Add garlic and cook 1 minute. Stir in flour. Slowly whisk in vegetable broth. Add miso, soy sauce, thyme, salt, and pepper. Simmer 5–7 minutes until thickened.

Make It Yours Ideas

Blend the entire gravy for a silky, creamy texture. Add a pinch of red pepper flakes.

Serve With

Portabella steaks, roasted vegetables, mashed potatoes, tofu, or rice bowls.

Coconut Pepper Gravy

Creamy, warm, and lightly spicy — a coconut-flavored gravy with black pepper heat. This one pairs beautifully with roasted vegetables, tofu steaks, rice bowls, and winter dishes.

Makes About 2 cups | Prep Time 5 minutes | Cook Time 10 minutes

Ingredients

1 tablespoon olive oil

½ cup finely diced onion

2 cloves garlic, minced

2 tablespoons flour

1 cup vegetable broth

1 cup canned coconut milk (full-fat or light)

1 teaspoon black pepper

½ teaspoon salt

¼ teaspoon turmeric (optional for color)

Directions

Warm olive oil in a saucepan. Add onion and cook 5 minutes. Add garlic and cook 1 minute. Add flour and stir to coat. Slowly whisk in vegetable broth and coconut milk. Add black pepper, salt, and turmeric. Simmer 8–10 minutes until creamy.

Make It Yours Ideas

Use half coconut milk and half cashew cream for a richer, thicker gravy.

Add a pinch of cayenne or crushed peppercorns.

Pairs With

Roasted cauliflower, tofu steaks, rice, mushrooms, sweet potatoes.

Rosemary Shallot Gravy

Elegant, aromatic, and herby — perfect for holiday plates, roasted dishes, or anytime you want a refined, restaurant-style gravy.

Makes About 2 cups | Prep Time 10 minutes | Cook Time 12 minutes

Ingredients

1 tablespoon vegan butter or olive oil

2 shallots, finely sliced

2 cloves garlic, minced

2 tablespoons flour

1 ½ cups vegetable broth

1 tablespoon soy sauce or coconut aminos

1 teaspoon fresh rosemary, finely chopped

½ teaspoon dried thyme

½ teaspoon salt

¼ teaspoon black pepper

Directions

Warm butter in a saucepan. Add shallots and cook 6–8 minutes, stirring often, until soft and fragrant. Add garlic and cook 1 minute. Stir in flour. Slowly whisk in broth. Add soy sauce, rosemary, thyme, salt, and pepper. Simmer 8–10 minutes until thickened.

Make It Yours Ideas

Add smoked paprika or black pepper.

Pairs With

Potatoes, mushrooms, vegetable roasts, tofu, chickpea cutlets.

5. Homemade "Packet-Style" Mixes

This section brings together simple, shelf-stable seasoning blends inspired by the convenience of store-bought packets—without the fillers, preservatives, or excess sodium. Each mix is designed to stir directly into sauces, gravies, dips, or marinades, giving you quick flavor boosts you can keep on hand for busy days. With just a few pantry ingredients, you can recreate the same ease of a packet while keeping everything aligned with your clean, plantsy-vegan cooking style.

- Ranch Seasoning Mix
- Dried Onion Soup Mix
- Brown Gravy Mix
- Simple Dry Rub for Vegetables and Tofu
- Preserved Lemon Herb Blend
- Dill Herb Seasoning Mix

Ranch Seasoning Mix

Perfect for gravies, dips, or dressings.

Makes About ½ cup

Ingredients

2 tablespoons dried parsley

1 tablespoon dried dill

1 tablespoon dried chives

1 tablespoon garlic powder

1 tablespoon onion powder

2 teaspoons dried onion flakes

2 teaspoons salt

1 teaspoon black pepper

Directions

Mix all ingredients. Store airtight up to 6 months.

Use

Add 1–2 tablespoons to gravies, dips, dressings, or roasted vegetables.

Dried Onion Soup Mix

Savory, comforting, slow-cooker friendly.

Makes About ½ cup

Ingredients

¼ cup dried minced onion

1 tablespoon onion powder

1 teaspoon garlic powder

1 teaspoon parsley

1 teaspoon celery seed

1 teaspoon salt

½ teaspoon black pepper

½ teaspoon smoked paprika (optional)

Directions

Mix ingredients and store airtight.

Use

Add 2 tablespoons to gravies, soups, mushrooms, roasts, or vegan meats.

Brown Gravy Mix

Packet-style convenience without the preservatives.

Makes About ½ cup

Ingredients

¼ cup flour

2 tablespoons nutritional yeast

1 tablespoon cornstarch

1 tablespoon onion powder

1 tablespoon garlic powder

1 teaspoon dried thyme

1 teaspoon paprika

1 teaspoon salt

½ teaspoon black pepper

Directions

Whisk to combine.

Use

Whisk 2 tablespoons into 1 cup broth to instantly thicken.

Simple Dry Rub for Vegetables and Tofu

A quick blend that adds warm, smoky flavor to tofu cutlets, roasted potatoes, chickpeas, eggplant, or mushrooms.

Makes about 3 tablespoons | Prep Time 2 minutes | Cook Time None

Ingredients

1 tablespoon smoked paprika

2 teaspoons brown sugar

1 teaspoon garlic powder

1 teaspoon onion powder

½ teaspoon ground cumin

½ teaspoon chili powder

¼ teaspoon black pepper

¼ teaspoon salt

Directions

1. Add all ingredients to a small bowl.
2. Stir the mixture until evenly blended.
3. Rub onto tofu or vegetables before baking, roasting, or grilling.

Preserved Lemon Herb Blend

Bright, salty, and intensely aromatic — preserved lemon adds a uniquely Mediterranean burst of flavor. This blend works as a finishing spoonful or a marinade booster.

Makes About 1½ cups | Prep Time 10 minutes

Ingredients

1 whole preserved lemon, rinsed and chopped (peel + pulp)

½ cup fresh parsley, finely chopped

¼ cup fresh mint, finely chopped

1 tablespoon olive oil

1 small garlic clove, minced

½ teaspoon black pepper

Directions

Stir chopped preserved lemon, parsley, mint, olive oil, garlic, and pepper in a bowl until well combined. Taste and adjust herbs or lemon as desired.

Make It Yours Ideas

Use only the lemon peel for a more delicate flavor.

Add a pinch of Aleppo pepper or smoked paprika.

Pairs With

Roasted potatoes, couscous, vegetables, tofu or grain bowls.

Dill Herb Seasoning Mix

A bright, savory, all-purpose herb mix that adds "fresh dill energy" to roasted vegetables, potatoes, tofu, grains, soups, and dips.

Makes About ½ cup | Prep Time 5 minutes

Ingredients

2 tablespoons dried dill
1 tablespoon dried parsley
1 tablespoon dried chives
2 teaspoons garlic powder
2 teaspoons onion powder
1 teaspoon fine sea salt
1 teaspoon dried oregano
½ teaspoon dried basil
½ teaspoon black pepper

Optional

½ teaspoon dried lemon zest for brightness
¼ teaspoon celery seed for savory depth
½ teaspoon nutritional yeast for umami
½ teaspoon paprika for a smoky flavor

Directions

1. Add all ingredients to a bowl or jar.
2. Mix or shake until fully combined.
3. Store in an airtight container for up to 6 months.

Make It Yours Ideas

Sprinkle on roasted potatoes, carrots, cauliflower, broccoli, or zucchini.

Season tofu, tempeh, or beans before cooking.

Mix into dips like vegan yogurt, mayo, or cream-style sauces.

Add to soups, stews, or chickpea salads.

Blend into vegan ranch-style dressings.

9. Condiment Sauces and Glazes

Everyday sauces built from pantry staples — simple, balanced, and made to enhance your favorite bowls, veggies, and mains.

This section uses everyday condiments as the building blocks for quick, reliable sauces and glazes. By combining familiar ingredients like mustard, ketchup, soy sauce, nut butters, and chili pastes with fresh aromatics and simple seasonings, you can create flavorful finishes that come together in minutes. These recipes are practical, versatile, and designed to help you transform basic pantry staples into sauces that work well for roasting, grilling, dipping, or drizzling over bowls and vegetables.

- Simple Mustard Sauce
- Sweet Chili Sauce
- Classic BBQ Sauce
- Peach BBQ Sause
- Mango BBQ Sauce
- Smoky Maple BBQ Sause
- Sweet and Smoky BBQ Sauce
- Korean-Style Gochujang BBQ Sause
- Classic Vegan Mayo (Base Recipe)
- Chipotle Mayo
- Chili Lime Mayo
- Garlic Herb Mayo
- Garlic Aioli Mayo
- Dijon Mayo
- Horseradish Mayo

Simple Mustard Sauce

A sharp, slightly creamy sauce that works well with roasted potatoes, tofu, tempeh, vegetable bowls, and warm grain salads.

Makes about ¾ cup | Prep Time 5 minutes | Cook Time 2 minutes

Ingredients

3 tablespoons Dijon mustard

2 tablespoons whole-grain mustard (optional for texture)

¼ cup water

2 tablespoons maple syrup

1 tablespoon apple cider vinegar

1 teaspoon olive oil

1 small clove garlic, grated

Salt and black pepper to taste

Directions

1. Add all of the ingredients to a small saucepan.
2. Stir the mixture until smooth.
3. Place the pan over low heat.
4. Warm 1–2 minutes until slightly thickened.
5. Taste and adjust vinegar, sweetness, or salt.

Sweet Chili Sauce

Bright, sticky, and lightly spicy — this homemade version skips the additives but keeps the classic sweet heat.

Makes About 2 cups | Prep Time 10 minutes | Cook Time 10 minutes

Ingredients

1 cup water

½ cup rice vinegar

½ cup coconut sugar

2 tablespoons tomato paste

2 cloves garlic, minced

1 tablespoon grated fresh ginger

1 tablespoon chili flakes or 2 fresh red chilies, minced

1 tablespoon cornstarch mixed with 2 tablespoons water

Directions

In a small saucepan, combine water, vinegar, sugar, tomato paste, garlic, ginger, and chili flakes. Bring to a boil over medium heat. Reduce to a simmer and cook 5 minutes.

Stir in the cornstarch slurry and whisk until thickened and glossy. Remove from heat and cool before storing.

Make It Yours Ideas

Add a splash of lime juice for brightness or a drizzle of sesame oil for richness. Use more chili flakes or add minced Thai chilies for extra fire.

Pairs With

Rice bowls, dumplings, spring rolls, or grilled vegetables.

Classic BBQ Sauce

A balanced, tangy barbecue sauce that works well for roasted vegetables, tofu slabs, cauliflower steaks, and grilled mushrooms.

Makes about 1 cup | Prep Time 5 minutes | Cook Time 10 minutes

Ingredients

1 cup tomato sauce

2 tablespoons maple syrup

1 tablespoon brown sugar

2 tablespoons apple cider vinegar

1 tablespoon tomato paste

1 teaspoon Dijon mustard

½ teaspoon smoked paprika

¼ teaspoon garlic powder

¼ teaspoon onion powder

⅛ teaspoon black pepper

Salt to taste

Directions

1. Add all ingredients to a saucepan.
2. Stir the mixture until combined.
3. Set the pan over medium heat.
4. Simmer 8–10 minutes until slightly thickened.
5. Taste and adjust sweetness, heat, or vinegar as desired.

Peach BBQ Sauce

A lightly sweet, tangy sauce that pairs well with tofu cutlets, mushrooms, roasted potatoes, and grilled summer vegetables.

Makes about 1 cup | Prep Time 10 minutes | Cook Time 12 minutes

Ingredients

1 cup diced peaches (fresh or frozen, thawed)

½ cup tomato sauce

2 tablespoons maple syrup

1 tablespoon apple cider vinegar

1 tablespoon soy sauce or tamari

1 teaspoon smoked paprika

½ teaspoon garlic powder

¼ teaspoon onion powder

¼ cup water

Salt to taste

Directions

1. Add all ingredients to a saucepan.
2. Stir until combined.
3. Bring the mixture to a low simmer.
4. Cook 10–12 minutes until the peaches soften.
5. Blend the mixture until smooth or leave slightly chunky.

Mango BBQ Sauce

A tropical-style barbecue sauce with gentle sweetness and mild heat, excellent for tofu, vegetable skewers, and roasted chickpeas.

Makes about 1 cup | Prep Time 10 minutes | Cook Time 10 minutes

Ingredients

1 cup diced mango (fresh or frozen, thawed)

½ cup tomato sauce

2 tablespoons maple syrup

1 tablespoon lime juice

1 tablespoon soy sauce or tamari

1 teaspoon chili powder

1 clove garlic

¼ cup water

Salt to taste

Directions

1. Add all ingredients to a saucepan.
2. Stir until combined.
3. Bring the mixture to a low simmer.
4. Cook 8–10 minutes.
5. Blend until smooth or leave slightly textured.

Smoky Maple BBQ Sauce

A sweeter, smoky version ideal for tofu, tempeh, or roasted chickpeas.

Makes about 1 cup | Prep Time 5 minutes | Cook Time 10 minutes

Ingredients

1 cup tomato sauce

3 tablespoons maple syrup

1 tablespoon soy sauce or tamari

1 tablespoon apple cider vinegar

1 teaspoon smoked paprika

½ teaspoon garlic powder

¼ teaspoon chili powder

1 tablespoon tomato paste

Salt to taste

Directions

1. Add all ingredients to a saucepan.
2. Whisk until smooth.
3. Bring to a low simmer.
4. Cook 8–10 minutes until slightly thickened.
5. Taste and adjust seasoning.

Sweet and Smoky BBQ Sauce

This from-scratch BBQ sauce balances sweetness, tang, and gentle smoke for a perfect all-purpose drizzle or marinade.

Makes About 2 cups | Prep Time 10 minutes | Cook Time 25 minutes

Ingredients

1 tablespoon olive oil

1 small onion, finely diced

2 cloves garlic, minced

1 can (6 ounces) tomato paste

1 cup water

¼ cup apple cider vinegar

¼ cup maple syrup

2 tablespoons molasses

1 tablespoon Dijon mustard

1 tablespoon smoked paprika

½ teaspoon salt

¼ teaspoon black pepper

¼ teaspoon cayenne (optional)

Directions

1. Heat olive oil in a saucepan over medium heat. Add onion and cook 5 minutes, until soft. Stir in garlic and cook 1 minute.
2. Add tomato paste, water, vinegar, maple syrup, molasses, mustard, paprika, salt, pepper, and cayenne.
3. Simmer uncovered 15–20 minutes, stirring occasionally, until thickened and glossy.

Make It Yours Ideas

Add 1 tablespoon tamari for savory depth

Add 1 teaspoon chili powder for more warmth.

Stir in chipotle paste or extra cayenne for a smoky kick.

Pairs With

BBQ cauliflower wings, lentil loaf, or grilled tempeh skewers.

Korean-Style Gochujang BBQ Sauce

A bold, sweet-spicy sauce that works well with tofu slabs, grilled mushrooms, roasted cauliflower, or sautéed vegetables.

Makes about 1 cup | Prep Time 5 minutes | Cook Time 8 minutes

Ingredients

2 tablespoons gochujang

2 tablespoons maple syrup

2 tablespoons soy sauce or tamari

1 tablespoon rice vinegar

1 tablespoon tomato paste

1 teaspoon grated garlic

1 teaspoon grated ginger

¼ cup water

Directions

1. Add all ingredients to a saucepan.
2. Stir until combined.
3. Place the pan over medium heat.
4. Bring the mixture to a low simmer.
5. Cook 6–8 minutes until slightly thickened.
6. Taste the sauce and adjust sweetness or heat as desired.

Classic Vegan Mayo (Base Recipe)

A simple, foolproof staple that serves as the base for every variation.

Makes About 2 cups | Prep Time 10 minutes

Ingredients

1 cup avocado oil

½ cup unsweetened soy milk or aquafaba

1 tablespoon lemon juice

1 teaspoon apple cider vinegar

½ teaspoon salt

1 teaspoon Dijon mustard

Directions

Blend all ingredients with an immersion blender or high-speed blender until thick and creamy. Chill at least 30 minutes before using.

Make It Yours Ideas

Swap lemon for lime or add a hint of maple for a mellow touch.

Stir in ¼ teaspoon cayenne or smoked paprika.

Pairs With

Sandwiches, wraps, burgers, or as a base for flavored mayos below.

Chipotle Mayo

Smoky, spicy, and full-bodied — perfect for tacos, roasted potatoes, or veggie burgers.

Makes About 2 cups | Prep Time 10 minutes

Ingredients

1 cup Classic Vegan Mayo (recipe above)

1–2 chipotle peppers in adobo, minced

1 tablespoon adobo sauce

1 teaspoon lime juice

¼ teaspoon smoked paprika

Directions

Whisk all ingredients together until smooth. Chill 30 minutes for flavors to deepen.

Make It Yours Ideas

Blend in a small roasted red pepper for extra sweetness.

Add a pinch of cayenne or hot sauce.

Pairs With

Tacos, sweet potato fries, grain bowls, or grilled corn.

Chili Lime Mayo

Bright and bold with a citrus kick — adds instant flavor to tacos, bowls, and sandwiches.

Makes About 2 cups | Prep Time 10 minutes

Ingredients

1 cup Classic Vegan Mayo (recipe above)

1 tablespoon lime juice

1 teaspoon lime zest

½ teaspoon chili powder

¼ teaspoon garlic powder

Pinch of salt

Directions

Whisk all ingredients until fully blended and smooth. Chill before serving.

Make It Yours Ideas

Add chopped cilantro or green onion for freshness.

Stir in minced jalapeño or hot sauce.

Pairs With

Cauliflower tacos, roasted vegetables, or grain bowls.

Garlic Herb Mayo

Creamy, aromatic, and herby — the perfect all-purpose spread.

Makes About 2 cups | Prep Time 10 minutes

Ingredients

1 cup Classic Vegan Mayo (recipe above)

1 tablespoon lemon juice

1 garlic clove, minced

1 tablespoon chopped parsley

1 teaspoon chopped dill

½ teaspoon salt

¼ teaspoon black pepper

Directions

Mix all ingredients until combined. Let rest 15 minutes before serving for flavors to meld.

Make It Yours Ideas

Swap herbs seasonally — basil and chives in spring, rosemary in fall.

Add a hint of Dijon mustard or horseradish.

Pairs With

Sandwiches, wraps or roasted potato wedges.

Garlic Aioli Mayo

Smooth, garlicky, and deeply flavorful — this vegan aioli adds a touch of richness to sandwiches, roasted vegetables, or grain bowls.

Makes About 2 cups | Prep Time 10 minutes

Ingredients

1 cup Classic Vegan Mayo (recipe above)

2–3 cloves garlic, minced or roasted

1 tablespoon lemon juice

1 teaspoon olive oil

¼ teaspoon salt

⅛ teaspoon black pepper

Directions

Blend or whisk all ingredients until fully incorporated and creamy. Chill for 30 minutes before serving to allow flavors to meld.

Make It Yours Ideas

For a milder aioli, roast the garlic cloves before blending.

Add a pinch of smoked paprika or chili flakes.

Pairs With

Grilled vegetables, veggie burgers, fries, or roasted potatoes.

Dijon Mayo

Tangy, sharp, and perfectly balanced — this Dijon mayo makes an ideal sandwich spread or salad dressing base.

Makes About 2 cups | Prep Time 10 minutes

Ingredients

1 cup Classic Vegan Mayo (recipe above)

1 tablespoon Dijon mustard

1 teaspoon lemon juice

½ teaspoon maple syrup

¼ teaspoon garlic powder

Pinch of salt and pepper

Directions

Whisk together all ingredients until smooth and creamy. Adjust lemon and mustard to taste.

Make It Yours Ideas

Add a small spoonful of capers or chopped herbs for a more complex flavor.

Stir in a little prepared horseradish or crushed black pepper.

Pairs With

Sandwiches, wraps, potato salad, or as a base for vinaigrettes.

Horseradish Mayo

Zesty and bold — a classic condiment with a vegan twist, perfect for sandwiches, grain bowls, and roasted vegetables.

Makes About 2 cups | Prep Time 10 minutes

Ingredients

1 cup Classic Vegan Mayo (recipe above)

1 tablespoon prepared horseradish (or more to taste)

1 teaspoon lemon juice

½ teaspoon Dijon mustard

¼ teaspoon salt

⅛ teaspoon black pepper

Directions

Combine all ingredients in a bowl and whisk until creamy and evenly blended. Taste and adjust seasoning as desired. Chill before serving.

Make It Yours Ideas

Add grated apple for sweetness and depth.

Mix in a pinch of cayenne for an extra kick.

Pairs With

Sandwiches, roasted root vegetables or as a dip for baked fries.

10. Mediterranean Sauces

Bright, bold, and rooted in simple ingredients — Mediterranean sauces bring together olive oil, fresh herbs, roasted peppers, citrus, garlic, and nuts to create deeply flavorful accents for bowls, vegetables, pastas, and breads.

These sauces celebrate balance: richness from tahini or nuts, brightness from lemon or vinegar, and savory depth from olives, capers, and herbs. Use them to elevate everyday plantsy meals with the sun-soaked flavors of the Mediterranean.

- Sidebar: About Mediterranean Sauces
- Romesco Sauce
- Mediterranean Olive and Herb Sauce
- Mediterranean Tomato Caper Sauce
- Lemon Tahini Mediterranean Drizzle
- Tomato Caper Garlic Sauce
- Herbed Yogurt Tahini Mediterranean Blend
- Muhammara (Roasted Red Pepper and Walnut Sauce)
- Lemon Garlic Gremolata
- Tzatziki Style Cucumber Yogurt
- Lemon Oregano Mediterranean Marinade
- Basil Walnut Pesto

Sidebar: About Mediterranean Sauces

Mediterranean sauces are built on simple ingredients layered with bold flavor. They typically include one or more of the following elements:

1. Olive Oil

The foundation of Mediterranean cooking — adds richness and depth.

2. Fresh Herbs

Parsley, basil, dill, mint, oregano, and rosemary bring brightness and aroma.

3. Citrus and Vinegars

Lemon juice, lemon zest, and red wine vinegar create acidity and lift.

4. Nuts and Seeds

Walnuts, almonds, pine nuts, tahini, and sometimes hazelnuts add body and creaminess.

5. Roasted Vegetables

Red peppers, tomatoes, and garlic contribute sweetness, smokiness, and umami.

6. Salty, Savory Accents

Olives, capers, and preserved lemon deepen complexity.

7. Warm Spice Notes

Smoked paprika, cumin, Aleppo pepper, and sumac create warmth without overpowering.

Together, these elements create sauces that are vibrant, balanced, and incredibly versatile — perfect for vegetables, bowls, pasta, breads, and plant-based proteins. This section brings those flavors home in simple, everyday ways.

Romesco Sauce

Bold, smoky, and deeply flavorful — perfect with vegetables, bowls, pasta, or crusty bread.

Romesco is one of the most beloved Mediterranean sauces — bold, smoky, nutty, and incredibly versatile. It originated in Tarragona, Spain, and was traditionally made by fishermen to serve with grilled seafood. Today, it's used on vegetables, potatoes, pasta, sandwiches, and dips.

Makes About 1 cup | Prep Time 10 minutes | Cook Time 10 minutes

Ingredients

2 large roasted red bell peppers (jarred, drained)
1 medium tomato, halved
3 cloves garlic
¼ cup raw almonds (or hazelnuts)
2 tablespoons tomato paste
2 tablespoons red wine vinegar
1 tablespoon olive oil
1 teaspoon smoked paprika
½ teaspoon salt
¼ teaspoon black pepper

Directions

Broil the tomato and garlic on a lined sheet until lightly charred — about 8–10 minutes. Toast almonds in a dry skillet until fragrant. Add roasted peppers, tomato, garlic, almonds, tomato paste, red wine vinegar, olive oil, smoked paprika, salt, and pepper to a blender. Blend until smooth and thick. Adjust seasoning to taste.

Make It Yours Ideas

Use hazelnuts for a deeper, richer, more traditional Spanish flavor.

Add ⅛ teaspoon cayenne or a pinch of chili flakes.

Pairs With - Roasted vegetables, potatoes, veggie patties, grain bowls, pasta or grilled tofu.

Mediterranean Olive and Herb Sauce

Rustic, savory, and deeply aromatic — a chopped olive-herb condiment that works as a sauce, spread, or finishing spoonful.

Makes About 2 cups | Prep Time 10 minutes

Ingredients

1 cup mixed olives, pitted and finely chopped

¼ cup olive oil

2 tablespoons red wine vinegar

2 tablespoons chopped fresh parsley

1 tablespoon chopped fresh basil

1 tablespoon capers, chopped

1 small garlic clove, minced

½ teaspoon lemon zest

½ teaspoon black pepper

Directions

Combine chopped olives, olive oil, vinegar, parsley, basil, capers, garlic, lemon zest, and pepper in a bowl. Stir until well mixed and glossy.

Make It Yours Ideas

Add chopped roasted red peppers or sun-dried tomatoes.

Stir in crushed red pepper flakes.

Pairs With

Pasta, bruschetta, salads, roasted vegetables, or grain bowls.

Mediterranean Tomato Caper Sauce

A savory, briny sauce that works well with roasted vegetables, pasta, tofu, and grain bowls.

Makes about 1 cup | Prep Time 10 minutes | Cook Time 10 minutes

Ingredients

1 tablespoon olive oil

2 cloves garlic, minced

1½ cups crushed tomatoes

2 tablespoons capers, drained

1 tablespoon tomato paste

½ teaspoon dried oregano

Black pepper to taste

Salt if needed

Directions

1. Heat the olive oil in a saucepan over medium heat.
2. Add the garlic and cook 1 minute.
3. Stir in the crushed tomatoes, capers, tomato paste, and oregano.
4. Simmer 8–10 minutes.
5. Taste and adjust salt or pepper.

Lemon Tahini Mediterranean Drizzle

Creamy, citrusy, and versatile — perfect for roasted vegetables, bowls, and salads.

Makes About 2 cups | Prep Time 5 minutes

Ingredients

½ cup tahini

½ cup water

¼ cup lemon juice

1 tablespoon olive oil

1 small garlic clove, grated

½ teaspoon salt

¼ teaspoon black pepper

Directions

Whisk tahini, water, lemon juice, olive oil, garlic, salt, and pepper until smooth and pourable. Add more water for a thinner drizzle.

Make It Yours Ideas

Add a spoonful of yogurt for a creamier finish.

Stir in smoked paprika or Aleppo pepper.

Pairs With

Roasted vegetables, falafel, bowls, salads.

Tomato Caper Garlic Sauce

Bright, savory, and Mediterranean through and through — excellent warm or at room temperature.

Makes About 2 cups | Prep Time 10 minutes   Cook Time 10 minutes

Ingredients

1 tablespoon olive oil

4 cloves garlic, sliced

3 medium tomatoes, chopped

2 tablespoons capers

2 tablespoons chopped fresh parsley

½ teaspoon salt

¼ teaspoon black pepper

Directions

Warm olive oil in a skillet. Add garlic and cook 1–2 minutes. Add tomatoes, capers, salt, and pepper. Simmer 7–10 minutes, until tomatoes break down slightly. Stir in parsley and remove from heat.

Make It Yours Ideas

Add olives for a heartier version.

Add crushed red pepper flakes.

Pairs With

Pasta, chickpeas, bruschetta, grilled vegetables.

Herbed Yogurt Tahini Mediterranean Blend

Creamy, herby, and cooling — a perfect contrast to roasted or spiced dishes.

Makes About 2 cups | Prep Time 5 minutes

Ingredients

1 cup vegan yogurt (coconut or cashew)

2 tablespoons tahini

1 tablespoon lemon juice

1 tablespoon olive oil

2 tablespoons chopped fresh dill or parsley

½ teaspoon garlic powder

½ teaspoon salt

¼ teaspoon black pepper

Directions

Mix yogurt, tahini, lemon juice, olive oil, dill, garlic powder, salt, and pepper until smooth. Chill before serving.

Make It Yours Ideas

Add cucumber for a tzatziki-inspired variation.

Add Aleppo pepper or za'atar.

Pairs With

Bowls, wraps, roasted potatoes, fresh vegetables.

Muhammara
(Roasted Pepper and Walnut Sauce)

Rich, smoky, and slightly sweet — a classic Middle Eastern/Mediterranean dip that also works beautifully as a sauce for bowls, roasted vegetables, and sandwiches.

Makes About 2 cups | Prep Time 10 minutes | Cook Time 10 minutes

Ingredients

2 large roasted red bell peppers (homemade or jarred, drained)

¾ cup walnuts, toasted

2 tablespoons tomato paste

2 tablespoons olive oil

1 tablespoon lemon juice

1 tablespoon pomegranate molasses (or 1 tablespoon balsamic vinegar + ½ teaspoon maple syrup)

1 small garlic clove

1 teaspoon smoked paprika

½ teaspoon salt

¼ teaspoon black pepper

Directions

Add roasted peppers, toasted walnuts, tomato paste, olive oil, lemon juice, pomegranate molasses, garlic, paprika, salt, and pepper to a blender. Blend until thick and smooth. Adjust seasoning to taste.

Make It Yours Ideas

Add 2–3 tablespoons breadcrumbs to thicken for a dip-style texture.

Blend in ⅛ teaspoon cayenne or chili flakes.

Pairs With - Pita, grain bowls, roasted vegetables, sandwiches, or grilled tofu.

Lemon Garlic Gremolata

Bright, fresh, and herby — the perfect finishing spoonful for vegetables, pasta, bowls, and roasted potatoes.

Makes About 1 cup | Prep Time 5 minutes

Ingredients

1 cup chopped fresh parsley

1 tablespoon grated lemon zest

2 cloves garlic, finely minced

2 tablespoons olive oil

¼ teaspoon salt

¼ teaspoon black pepper

Directions

Combine parsley, lemon zest, garlic, olive oil, salt, and pepper in a bowl. Stir until evenly mixed.

Make It Yours Ideas

Add chopped basil or mint for a softer, aromatic variation.

Include a pinch of crushed red pepper.

Pairs With

Roasted potatoes, pasta, grain bowls, grilled vegetables, soups.

Tzatziki Style Cucumber Yogurt

Cool, creamy, and refreshing — this dairy-free version of the classic Greek sauce brings brightness and balance to bowls, wraps, roasted vegetables, and grilled tofu.

Makes About 2 cups | Prep Time 10 minutes

Ingredients

1 ½ cups vegan yogurt (coconut or cashew)

1 cup finely grated cucumber (peeled or unpeeled)

1 tablespoon lemon juice

1 tablespoon olive oil

1 garlic clove, finely grated

2 tablespoons chopped fresh dill

½ teaspoon salt

¼ teaspoon black pepper

Directions

Squeeze excess water from the grated cucumber using a towel or paper towels. Add cucumber to a bowl with yogurt, lemon juice, olive oil, garlic, dill, salt, and pepper. Stir until smooth and well combined. Chill before serving.

Make It Yours Ideas

Use mint instead of dill for a softer flavor.

Add a pinch of Aleppo pepper or smoked paprika.

Pairs With

Falafel, vegetable wraps, grain bowls, potatoes, or grilled tofu.

Lemon Oregano Mediterranean Marinade

Bright, zesty, and herby — perfect for marinating tofu, vegetables, chickpeas, or for drizzling over bowls and salads.

Makes About 2 cups | Prep Time 5 minutes

Ingredients

½ cup olive oil

¼ cup lemon juice

1 tablespoon lemon zest

2 tablespoons red wine vinegar

2 garlic cloves, minced

1 tablespoon dried oregano

1 teaspoon Dijon mustard

1 teaspoon salt

½ teaspoon black pepper

Directions

Whisk olive oil, lemon juice, lemon zest, vinegar, garlic, oregano, mustard, salt, and pepper until emulsified. Use immediately or refrigerate.

Make It Yours Ideas

Add chopped fresh parsley or basil for a more aromatic finish.

Stir in crushed red pepper flakes or a pinch of cumin.

Pairs With

Roasted vegetables, chickpeas, tofu, potatoes, or grain bowls.

Basil Walnut Pesto

Bright, aromatic, and full of Mediterranean character — this pesto uses walnuts (instead of pine nuts) for a richer, earthier flavor and a beautifully creamy texture.

Makes About 2 cups | Prep Time 10 minutes

Ingredients

3 cups fresh basil leaves, loosely packed

½ cup walnuts, lightly toasted

2 cloves garlic

¼ cup nutritional yeast

½ cup olive oil

2 tablespoons lemon juice

½ teaspoon salt

¼ teaspoon black pepper

Directions

Add basil, walnuts, garlic, nutritional yeast, olive oil, lemon juice, salt, and pepper to a food processor. Blend until smooth or leave slightly textured. Adjust seasoning to taste.

Make It Yours Ideas

Replace half the basil with parsley or spinach for a milder, softer flavor.

Add a pinch of crushed red pepper flakes.

Pairs With

Pasta, roasted vegetables, toast, sandwiches, grain bowls, or chickpeas.

11. Everyday Sauces and Glazes

This section gathers quick, dependable sauces and glazes you can use throughout the week to add flavor without extra effort. From bright, citrusy blends to creamy herb sauces and simple sweet-savory glazes, these recipes rely on familiar ingredients and straightforward. Whether you need a dip, a drizzle, a bowl topper, or a finishing touch for tofu or vegetables, these everyday options are designed to give you reliable results and flexible flavor in minutes.

- Peanut Lime Sauce
- Miso Tahini Sauce
- Ginger Scallion Sauce
- Dill Garlic Sauce
- Creamy Dill Sauce
- Creamy Dill Sauce with Chopped Pickles
- Teriyaki Sauce
- Pineapple Ginger Teriyaki Sauce
- Teriyaki Glaze
- Maple Mustard Glaze
- Brown Sugar Glaze
- Maple Chipotle Glaze

Peanut Lime Sauce

A creamy, tangy sauce ideal for tofu bowls, noodles, roasted broccoli, and vegetable wraps.

Makes about 1 cup | Prep Time 5 minutes | Cook Time None

Ingredients

¼ cup creamy peanut butter

2 tablespoons lime juice

2 tablespoons soy sauce or tamari

1 tablespoon maple syrup

1 tablespoon water

1 teaspoon grated fresh ginger

1 small clove garlic, grated

Red pepper flakes to taste

Directions

1. Add peanut butter, lime juice, soy sauce, maple syrup, and water to a bowl.
2. Whisk until smooth.
3. Stir in ginger, garlic, and red pepper flakes.
4. Taste and adjust lime or sweetness.

Miso Tahini Sauce

A savory, umami-rich sauce that works well with roasted vegetables, grain bowls, soups, and tofu.

Makes about ¾ cup | Prep Time 5 minutes | Cook Time None

Ingredients

2 tablespoons tahini

1 tablespoon white miso paste

1 tablespoon lemon juice

1 tablespoon maple syrup

2 tablespoons water

1 small clove garlic, grated

Black pepper to taste

Directions

1. Add tahini, miso, lemon juice, maple syrup, and water to a bowl.
2. Whisk until smooth.
3. Add garlic and black pepper.
4. Adjust water to thin if needed.

Ginger Scallion Sauce

A fragrant, all-purpose sauce that works well with tofu, rice bowls, noodles, and roasted vegetables.

Makes about ¾ cup | Prep Time 10 minutes | Cook Time 2 minutes

Ingredients

4 scallions, finely minced

2 tablespoons grated fresh ginger

¼ cup avocado oil

1 tablespoon soy sauce or tamari

1 tablespoon rice vinegar

½ teaspoon salt

Black pepper to taste

Directions

1. Add scallions, ginger, salt, and black pepper to a heat-safe bowl.
2. Heat the oil in a small saucepan until warm.
3. Pour the warm oil over the scallion mixture.
4. Stir in the soy sauce and vinegar.
5. Taste and adjust salt.

Dill Garlic Sauce

A savory, garlicky, herb-packed sauce perfect for potatoes, pasta, roasted vegetables, tofu, and Mediterranean-style bowls. This is a pourable sauce with a creamy texture.

Makes About 1 cup | Prep Time 10 minutes | Cook Time None

Ingredients

½ cup plain unsweetened vegan yogurt *or* blended silken tofu

¼ cup olive oil

2 tablespoons lemon juice

1 tablespoon white wine vinegar

2 cloves garlic, grated

2–3 tablespoons fresh dill, finely chopped

1 tablespoon dried chives *or* 2 tablespoons fresh

¼ teaspoon fine sea salt

Black pepper to taste

1 tablespoon tahini or cashew butter (optional, for richness)

Zest of ½ lemon (optional)

Directions

1. Add the vegan yogurt, olive oil, lemon juice, vinegar, and grated garlic to a bowl and whisk until smooth.
2. Add the dill, chives, salt, and pepper.
3. Whisk until creamy.
4. Add tahini or cashew butter, if using, to thicken. Adjust lemon or salt to taste.

Make It Yours Ideas

Add a splash of pickle brine for a tangy garlic-dill finish.

Add nutritional yeast for a mild cheesy note.

Add a small, minced jalapeño for heat.

Serving Ideas

Drizzle over roasted or boiled potatoes.

Spoon over pasta or warm grains.

Use as a dressing for Mediterranean bowls.

Serve with roasted cauliflower, broccoli, carrots or zucchini.

Use as a sauce for tofu steaks or cutlets.

Creamy Dill Sauce

Bright, tangy, and herby, this sauce is smooth and versatile. It's perfect for roasted vegetables, baked potatoes, grain bowls, tofu, salads, and wraps.

Makes about 1 cup | Prep time: 10 minutes | Cook time: None

Ingredients

½ cup plain unsweetened vegan yogurt or silken tofu

¼ cup unsweetened plant milk

2 tablespoons lemon juice

1 tablespoon olive oil

1 tablespoon Dijon mustard

1 tablespoon maple syrup

1 small clove garlic, grated or minced

2–3 tablespoons finely chopped fresh dill

¼ teaspoon fine sea salt, plus more to taste

Black pepper to taste

1 tablespoon vegan mayo (adds smooth thickness)

1 tablespoon cashew butter (whisk until fully blended for creaminess)

Directions

1. Add the vegan yogurt or silken tofu, plant milk, lemon juice, olive oil, Dijon mustard, maple syrup, garlic, vegan mayo, and cashew butter to a bowl and whisk until smooth.
2. Add the fresh dill, salt, and black pepper.
3. Stir until evenly combined.
4. Adjust seasoning as needed.
5. Refrigerate for 20–30 minutes to allow the dill flavor to deepen.

Creamy Dill Sauce with Chopped Pickles

This sauce picks up finely chopped pickles for a tangy, pickle sauce perfect for roasted potatoes, veggie burgers, sandwiches, wraps, bowls, and tofu nuggets.

Makes About 1¼ cups | Prep Time 10 minutes

Ingredients

Use the base Dill Sauce recipe and add:

2–3 tablespoons finely chopped dill pickles

1–2 teaspoons pickle brine (start with 1 teaspoon and adjust)

1 tablespoon finely chopped fresh parsley (optional)

½ teaspoon capers, minced (optional)

Directions

1. Prepare the base Dill Sauce according to the directions.
2. Stir in the chopped pickles and pickle brine.
3. Add parsley or capers if using.
4. Add extra brine for a sharper pickle note.
5. Chill for 20 minutes before serving.

Serving Ideas

Drizzle over baked or air-fried sweet potatoes.

Spoon onto veggie burgers or wraps.

Serve with roasted carrots, cauliflower, or zucchini.

Use as a dip for potatoes, chickpea patties or tofu.

Add to quinoa or grain bowls.

Teriyaki Sauce

A simple, lightly sweet teriyaki that works well as a marinade or finishing sauce.

Makes about ¾ cup | Prep Time 5 minutes | Cook Time 8 minutes

Ingredients

¼ cup soy sauce or tamari

¼ cup water

2 tablespoons maple syrup

1 tablespoon rice vinegar

1 tablespoon grated fresh ginger

1 clove garlic, grated

1 teaspoon sesame oil

1 tablespoon cornstarch mixed with 2 tablespoons water

Directions

1. Add soy sauce, water, maple syrup, vinegar, ginger, garlic, and sesame oil to a saucepan.
2. Stir to combine.
3. Set the pan over medium heat.
4. Add the cornstarch slurry.
5. Whisk until the mixture thickens, about 2–3 minutes.
6. Remove the pan from the heat when the sauce coats a spoon.

Pineapple Ginger Teriyaki Sauce

A fruity twist on classic teriyaki that creates a glossy, sweet sauce perfect for tofu cubes, vegetable stir-fries and roasted chickpeas.

Makes about 1 cup | Prep Time 5 minutes | Cook Time 8 minutes

Ingredients

½ cup pineapple juice

¼ cup soy sauce or tamari

2 tablespoons maple syrup

1 tablespoon rice vinegar

1 tablespoon grated fresh ginger

1 clove garlic, grated

1 teaspoon sesame oil

1 tablespoon cornstarch mixed with 2 tablespoons water

Directions

1. Add pineapple juice, soy sauce, maple syrup, vinegar, ginger, garlic, and sesame oil to a saucepan.
2. Stir to combine.
3. Set the pan over medium heat.
4. Add the cornstarch slurry.
5. Whisk until thick and glossy.
6. Remove from heat when the sauce coats a spoon.

Teriyaki Glaze

A glossy, umami-rich glaze made from simple ingredients — perfect for stir-fries, tofu, or roasted vegetables.

Makes About 2 cups | Prep Time 5 minutes | Cook Time 10 minutes

Ingredients

½ cup soy sauce or tamari

½ cup water

¼ cup maple syrup or coconut sugar

2 tablespoons rice vinegar

1 tablespoon grated fresh ginger

1 garlic clove, minced

1 tablespoon cornstarch mixed with 2 tablespoons water

Directions

In a small saucepan, combine soy sauce, water, maple syrup, vinegar, ginger, and garlic. Bring to a gentle boil. Stir in the cornstarch slurry and whisk until the sauce thickens and becomes glossy, about 2–3 minutes. Remove from heat.

Make It Yours Ideas

Add 1 teaspoon sesame oil or 1 tablespoon orange juice for a citrus note.

Stir in chili flakes or a few drops of hot sauce.

Pairs With

Stir-fried veggies, tofu, tempeh, or rice bowls.

Maple Mustard Glaze

Sweet, tangy, and balanced — this glaze turns simple roasted vegetables or tofu into something special.

Makes About 2 cups | Prep Time 5 minutes | Cook Time 5 minutes

Ingredients

¼ cup Dijon mustard

¼ cup whole-grain mustard

⅓ cup maple syrup

2 tablespoons apple cider vinegar

2 tablespoons olive oil

½ teaspoon salt

¼ teaspoon black pepper

Directions

Whisk all ingredients in a small saucepan. Warm over medium heat for 3–5 minutes until slightly thickened and glossy.

Make It Yours Ideas

Add a spoonful of minced fresh herbs like rosemary or thyme for depth.

Stir in ¼ teaspoon cayenne or 1 teaspoon horseradish for zip.

Pairs With

Roasted carrots, tempeh, grilled tofu, or grain bowls.

Brown Sugar Glaze

A glossy, sweet glaze that works well with mushrooms, tofu, roasted carrots, and baked sweet potatoes.

Makes about ½ cup | Prep Time 5 minutes | Cook Time 5 minutes

Ingredients

3 tablespoons brown sugar

2 tablespoons maple syrup

1 tablespoon soy sauce or tamari

1 tablespoon apple cider vinegar

¼ teaspoon smoked paprika

¼ cup water

Directions

1. Add all ingredients to a small saucepan.
2. Whisk until combined.
3. Simmer 4–5 minutes over medium heat until slightly thickened.
4. Taste and adjust sweetness or vinegar.

Maple Chipotle Glaze

A sweet, smoky glaze ideal for tofu slabs, roasted carrots, sweet potatoes, and cauliflower steaks.

Makes about ½ cup | Prep Time 5 minutes | Cook Time 3 minutes

Ingredients

¼ cup maple syrup

1 tablespoon tomato paste

1 tablespoon soy sauce or tamari

1 teaspoon chipotle powder

1 teaspoon apple cider vinegar

1 tablespoon water

Directions

1. Add all ingredients to a small saucepan.
2. Whisk until smooth.
3. Warm 2–3 minutes over low heat until slightly thickened.
4. Brush onto tofu or vegetables before roasting or grilling.

12. Marinades

This section highlights simple marinades that infuse tofu, vegetables, and plant-based proteins with bright, balanced flavor. Each recipe uses everyday pantry staples—citrus, herbs, soy sauce, aromatics, and a touch of sweetness—to tenderize ingredients and help them cook up with deeper taste and better texture. Whether you're preparing a quick weeknight meal or planning ahead for batch cooking, these marinades make it easy to add dimension without extra work.

How to Use These Marinades and Tips for Best Results

For best flavor, let tofu, vegetables, or plant-based proteins marinate for at least 20–30 minutes, or up to several hours if you have the time. Tofu benefits from being pressed first so it can absorb more liquid, while vegetables like mushrooms, zucchini, peppers, and onions take on flavor quickly with shorter marinating times. If you plan to roast or grill, reserve a small amount of marinade to brush on during cooking for added caramelization. These marinades are designed to be flexible—use them for sheet-pan meals, stir-fries, grilling, air-frying, or batch-cooking components for the week. A little time in a flavorful marinade helps ingredients cook up with deeper taste and better texture.

- Soy Ginger Marinade
- Sweet Garlic Marinade
- Sesame Orange Marinade
- Chili Lime Marinade
- Lemon Mustard Herb Marinade
- Lemon Dill Marinade

Soy Ginger Marinade

A bright, savory marinade for tofu, tempeh, vegetables, or mushrooms.

Makes about ½ cup | Prep Time 5 minutes | Cook Time None

Ingredients

¼ cup soy sauce or tamari

2 tablespoons rice vinegar

1 tablespoon maple syrup

1 tablespoon grated fresh ginger

1 small clove garlic, grated

1 teaspoon sesame oil

2 tablespoons water

Black pepper to taste

Directions

1. Add all ingredients to a bowl.
2. Stir the mixture until smooth.
3. Pour the marinade over tofu or vegetables.
4. Let the mixture rest at least 20 minutes before cooking.

Sweet Garlic Marinade

Good for tofu cutlets, roasted cauliflower or portabella mushrooms.

Makes about ½ cup | Prep Time 5 minutes | Cook Time None

Ingredients

3 tablespoons soy sauce or tamari

2 tablespoons maple syrup

1 tablespoon lemon juice

1 tablespoon olive oil

1 clove garlic, grated

1 tablespoon water

Black pepper to taste

Directions

1. Add all ingredients to a bowl.
2. Whisk until smooth.
3. Use immediately or refrigerate up to 3 days.

Sesame Orange Marinade

A lightly sweet, citrusy marinade that works well with tofu, tempeh, broccoli, mushrooms, and roasted carrots.

Makes about ½ cup | Prep Time 5 minutes | Cook Time None

Ingredients

¼ cup fresh-squeezed orange juice

2 tablespoons soy sauce or tamari

1 tablespoon rice vinegar

1 tablespoon maple syrup

1 teaspoon sesame oil

1 teaspoon grated fresh ginger

1 clove garlic, grated

1 tablespoon water

Directions

1. Add all ingredients to a bowl.
2. Whisk until smooth.
3. Pour over tofu or vegetables and let rest at least 20 minutes.

Chili Lime Marinade

A crisp, spicy marinade that brightens tofu, tempeh, grilled vegetables, and roasted cauliflower.

Makes about ½ cup | Prep Time 5 minutes | Cook Time None

Ingredients

¼ cup lime juice

2 tablespoons olive oil

1 tablespoon maple syrup

1 tablespoon soy sauce or tamari

1 teaspoon chili powder

½ teaspoon smoked paprika

1 clove garlic, grated

1 tablespoon water

Salt and black pepper to taste

Directions

1. Add all ingredients to a bowl.
2. Whisk until smooth.
3. Marinate tofu or vegetables at least 20 minutes before cooking.

Lemon Mustard Herb Marinade

Bright and tangy, this marinade is ideal for tofu, tempeh, asparagus, zucchini, or roasted chickpeas.

Makes about ½ cup | Prep Time 5 minutes | Cook Time None

Ingredients

¼ cup lemon juice

2 tablespoons olive oil

1 tablespoon maple syrup

1 tablespoon Dijon mustard

1 teaspoon dried oregano or parsley

1 small clove garlic, grated

1 tablespoon water

Salt and black pepper to taste

Directions

1. Add all ingredients to a bowl.
2. Whisk until smooth.
3. Use immediately or marinate tofu or vegetables 20–30 minutes.

Lemon Dill Marinade

Bright, herby, and versatile, this marinade works beautifully with tofu, tempeh, vegetables, potatoes, roasted chickpeas, and as a quick drizzle for bowls and salads.

Makes about ¾ cup | Prep time: 10 minutes | Cook time: None

Ingredients

¼ cup olive oil

3 tablespoons lemon juice

2 tablespoons apple cider vinegar

1 tablespoon maple syrup

1 tablespoon Dijon mustard

1 clove garlic, minced

2–3 tablespoons fresh dill, chopped

½ teaspoon dried oregano

¼ teaspoon fine sea salt

Black pepper to taste

Zest of ½ lemon

1 teaspoon pickle brine

1–2 tablespoons water

Directions

Add the olive oil, lemon juice, vinegar, maple syrup, Dijon mustard, garlic, dill, oregano, salt, black pepper, lemon zest, pickle brine, and water to a bowl or jar. Whisk or shake until fully emulsified. Adjust seasoning as needed.

Use It For

Tofu - Marinate slices, cubes, or crumbles for 20–30 minutes.

Vegetables - Toss zucchini, potatoes, carrots, cauliflower, or green beans before roasting.

Chickpeas - Marinate before air-frying or roasting.

Bowls - Use as a drizzle over grains, greens, and veggies.

13. Vinaigrettes

Bright, balanced, and versatile — the finishing touches that pull a plate together and bring every bite to life.

This section features light, balanced dressings that rely on simple pantry ingredients to brighten salads, vegetables, bowls, and grain dishes. Each vinaigrette blends acidity, sweetness, and aromatics to create a clean, versatile finish that can be whisked together in minutes. Whether you prefer citrus-flavored, maple-sweetened, or herb-driven flavors, these recipes offer dependable options that bring fresh dimension to everyday meals.

How to Adjust Flavor and Best Ways to Use These Vinaigrettes

Vinaigrettes are easy to tailor to your preferred balance of acidity, sweetness, and richness. To mellow sharpness, whisk in a splash of maple syrup or a bit more oil. For a brighter, tangier finish, add an extra teaspoon of vinegar or citrus juice. If the dressing feels too thin, blend or whisk in a small amount of mustard or tahini to help it emulsify; if it's too thick, loosen it with a teaspoon of water. These vinaigrettes work well on leafy salads, grain bowls, roasted vegetables, or as a quick marinade for tofu or chickpeas. They're designed to bring freshness and clarity to everyday meals with just a few simple adjustments.

- Classic Lemon Vinaigrette
- Apple Cider Maple Dressing
- Balsamic Dijon Vinaigrette
- Orange Tahini Vinaigrette
- Mediterranean Herb Vinaigrette

Classic Lemon Vinaigrette

Clean, zesty, and endlessly useful, this simple vinaigrette is your go-to for greens, grain bowls, or roasted vegetables.

Makes About 2 cups | Prep Time 10 minutes

Ingredients

½ cup fresh lemon juice (about 4 lemons)

¾ cup olive oil

2 teaspoons Dijon mustard

1 tablespoon maple syrup

1 small garlic clove, minced

½ teaspoon salt

¼ teaspoon black pepper

Directions

Whisk all ingredients in a bowl or shake together in a sealed jar until emulsified. Taste and adjust seasoning as needed.

Make It Yours Ideas

Add chopped fresh herbs like parsley or basil for a green vinaigrette.

Include a pinch of chili flakes or a few drops of hot sauce.

Pairs With

Mixed greens, lentil salads, quinoa bowls, or roasted asparagus.

Apple Cider Maple Dressing

A lightly sweet dressing that pairs crisp apple cider tang with the richness of olive oil and the warmth of maple.

Makes About 2 cups | Prep Time 10 minutes

Ingredients

½ cup apple cider vinegar

¾ cup olive oil

2 tablespoons maple syrup

1 tablespoon Dijon mustard

1 teaspoon minced shallot

½ teaspoon salt

¼ teaspoon black pepper

Directions

Whisk all ingredients together until smooth and creamy. Store in the refrigerator up to one week; shake before using.

Make It Yours Ideas

Stir in a spoonful of tahini or almond butter for a creamy texture.

Add a pinch of cinnamon or nutmeg for autumn-inspired flavor.

Pairs With

Kale salads, roasted root vegetables or apple-quinoa bowls.

Balsamic Dijon Vinaigrette

A classic, slightly tangy dressing that works for everything from hearty salads to grilled vegetables.

Makes About 2 cups | Prep Time 10 minutes

Ingredients

½ cup balsamic vinegar

¾ cup olive oil

1 tablespoon Dijon mustard

1 tablespoon maple syrup or agave

1 clove garlic, minced

½ teaspoon salt

¼ teaspoon black pepper

Directions

Whisk vinegar, mustard, maple syrup, and garlic together. Slowly whisk in olive oil until emulsified. Season with salt and pepper.

Make It Yours Ideas

Replace half the balsamic with red wine vinegar for a lighter flavor.

Add crushed red pepper flakes or a dash of smoked paprika.

Pairs With

Spinach salads, roasted tomatoes, or grain bowls with lentils.

Orange Tahini Vinaigrette

Bright, creamy, and citrusy — a Middle Eastern-inspired dressing that adds richness and zing to bowls and greens.

Makes About 2 cups | Prep Time 10 minutes

Ingredients

½ cup fresh orange juice (1 large orange)

¼ cup lemon juice

¼ cup tahini

¼ cup olive oil

2 tablespoons maple syrup

1 garlic clove, minced

½ teaspoon salt

¼ teaspoon black pepper

Directions

Whisk orange juice, lemon juice, tahini, olive oil, maple syrup, garlic, salt, and pepper together until smooth and creamy. Thin with a tablespoon of water if needed.

Make It Yours Ideas

Add grated ginger or a dash of cinnamon for warmth.

Stir in chili flakes for a hint of heat.

Pairs With

Grain bowls, chickpea salads or roasted carrots.

Mediterranean Herb Vinaigrette

Herbaceous, tangy, and full of fresh flavor — this vinaigrette brings a coastal flair to any meal.

Makes About 2 cups | Prep Time 10 minutes

Ingredients

½ cup red wine vinegar

¾ cup olive oil

1 tablespoon lemon juice

1 teaspoon Dijon mustard

1 teaspoon maple syrup

1 tablespoon finely chopped fresh oregano (or 1 teaspoon dried)

1 tablespoon chopped fresh basil or parsley

1 clove garlic, minced

½ teaspoon salt

¼ teaspoon black pepper

Directions

Whisk vinegar, lemon juice, mustard, and maple syrup together. Add herbs, garlic, salt, and pepper. Slowly whisk in olive oil until emulsified.

Make It Yours Ideas

Add 1 tablespoon chopped sun-dried tomatoes for extra depth.

Mix in a pinch of chili flakes or smoked paprika.

Pairs With

Greek-style salads, couscous, roasted chickpeas or grilled eggplant.

14. Creamy Dressings

Smooth, rich, and full of plant-based goodness — these dressings double as dips and drizzles to elevate every meal.

This section brings together smooth, rich dressings made from wholesome, plant-based ingredients that deliver both texture and flavor. These recipes blend nuts, tofu, yogurt alternatives, herbs, and citrus into versatile sauces that work as dips, drizzles, and bowl toppers. Whether you're looking for something bright and tangy, herby, smoky, or ginger-spiced, these creamy options offer great ways to add body and balanced flavor to everyday meals.

How to Adjust Thickness and Best Ways to Use These Dressings

Each dressing in this section can be easily adjusted to suit how you plan to use it. For a thinner, pourable consistency, whisk in a teaspoon or two of water, plant milk, or citrus juice until it reaches the texture you like. For a thicker dip-style version, reduce the liquid slightly or blend in more cashews, tofu, or avocado. These creamy dressings are versatile—use them to top salads, grain bowls, and roasted vegetables, spoon them over baked potatoes or tacos, or serve them as dips for fresh vegetables, cauliflower wings, or plant-based protein. They are designed to adapt to everyday meals and add flavor without extra effort.

- Cashew Ranch Dressing
- Tofu Caesar Dressing
- Avocado Lime Dressing
- Greek Yogurt Dill Dressing
- Chipotle Cream Dressing
- Carrot Ginger Dressing
- Herb Tahini Dressing

Cashew Ranch Dressing

A classic ranch made plantsy — creamy, tangy, and herbed, with cashews taking the place of dairy.

Makes About 2 cups | Prep Time 10 minutes | Soak time: 30 minutes

Ingredients

1 cup raw cashews, soaked 30 minutes in hot water

¾ cup water

2 tablespoons lemon juice

1 tablespoon apple cider vinegar

1 garlic clove

1 teaspoon onion powder

½ teaspoon salt

¼ teaspoon black pepper

1 tablespoon chopped fresh dill

1 tablespoon chopped fresh parsley

1 teaspoon chopped chives

Directions

Blend soaked cashews, water, lemon juice, vinegar, garlic, onion powder, salt, and pepper until smooth. Stir in fresh herbs by hand. Chill at least 30 minutes before serving.

Make It Yours Ideas

Swap herbs for your favorites — basil or cilantro give it a new twist.

Add a dash of smoked paprika or cayenne.

Pairs With

Salads, roasted potatoes, veggie wraps, or cauliflower wings.

Tofu Caesar Dressing

Creamy, tangy, and garlicky — this Caesar keeps the traditional boldness without any dairy or eggs.

Makes About 2 cups | Prep Time 10 minutes

Ingredients

1 package (12 ounces) silken tofu, drained

3 tablespoons lemon juice

2 tablespoons olive oil

1 tablespoon Dijon mustard

1 tablespoon capers with a bit of brine

1 garlic clove

2 tablespoons nutritional yeast

½ teaspoon salt and ¼ teaspoon black pepper

Directions

Blend all ingredients until completely smooth and creamy. Chill for at least 30 minutes to let flavors deepen.

Make It Yours Ideas

Add 1 tablespoon vegan Worcestershire sauce for a traditional Caesar bite.

Blend in extra black pepper or a pinch of chili flakes.

Pairs With

Romaine salads, roasted chickpeas, or grilled tofu.

Avocado Lime Dressing

Bright and creamy, this dressing brings freshness to tacos, salads, and bowls.

Makes About 2 cups | Prep Time 10 minutes

Ingredients

1 ripe avocado

¼ cup olive oil

¼ cup water (more as needed to thin)

2 tablespoons lime juice

1 tablespoon apple cider vinegar

1 garlic clove

½ teaspoon salt

¼ teaspoon black pepper

1 tablespoon chopped cilantro (optional)

Directions

Blend all ingredients until smooth. Add more water if needed for desired consistency. Chill before serving.

Make It Yours Ideas

Add 1 tablespoon vegan yogurt for extra tang.

Blend in a jalapeño or a pinch of cayenne.

Pairs With

Tacos, burrito bowls, grilled corn, or roasted sweet potatoes.

Greek Yogurt Dill Dressing

Light, tangy, and refreshing — perfect for Mediterranean-style salads or wraps.

Makes About 2 cups | Prep Time 10 minutes

Ingredients

1½ cups unsweetened vegan yogurt (coconut or almond-based)

1 tablespoon lemon juice

1 tablespoon olive oil

1 clove garlic, minced

2 tablespoons chopped fresh dill

½ teaspoon salt

¼ teaspoon black pepper

Directions

Whisk all ingredients in a bowl until smooth. Chill at least 15 minutes before serving.

Make It Yours Ideas

Add grated cucumber for a tzatziki-style variation.

Add ¼ teaspoon ground cumin or smoked paprika.

Pairs With

Mediterranean salads, falafel wraps or roasted chickpeas.

Chipotle Cream Dressing

Smoky, spicy, and slightly sweet — a bold dressing that brings life to any meal.

Makes About 2 cups | Prep Time 10 minutes

Ingredients

1 cup raw cashews, soaked 30 minutes

¾ cup water

1 tablespoon lemon juice

1 tablespoon maple syrup

1 tablespoon tomato paste

1–2 chipotle peppers in adobo sauce (adjust to heat level)

1 garlic clove

½ teaspoon salt

Directions

Blend all ingredients until smooth and creamy. Adjust seasoning to taste and thin with water as needed.

Make It Yours Ideas

Add a splash of lime juice for brightness.

Include an extra chipotle pepper or a spoonful of adobo sauce.

Pairs With

Grain bowls, tacos, roasted vegetables, or sandwiches.

Carrot Ginger Dressing

A bright, smooth dressing that pairs well with salads, grain bowls, tofu, and roasted vegetables.

Makes about 1 cup | Prep Time 10 minutes | Cook Time 5 minutes

Ingredients

1 cup diced carrots

2 tablespoons rice vinegar

1 tablespoon soy sauce or tamari

1 tablespoon maple syrup

1 tablespoon grated fresh ginger

1 tablespoon olive oil

¼ cup water

Directions

1. Add carrots to a small saucepan.
2. Cover with water and simmer 5 minutes.
3. Drain the carrots.
4. Add carrots, vinegar, soy sauce, maple syrup, ginger, olive oil, and water to a blender.
5. Blend until smooth.
6. Add more water if needed to adjust thickness.

Herb Tahini Dressing

A creamy, herb-rich dressing perfect for bowls, salads, roasted vegetables, and chickpeas.

Makes about ¾ cup | Prep Time 5 minutes | Cook Time None

Ingredients

¼ cup tahini

3 tablespoons lemon juice

2 tablespoons water

1 tablespoon chopped parsley

1 tablespoon chopped cilantro

1 clove garlic, grated

Salt and black pepper to taste

Directions

1. Add tahini, lemon juice, and water to a bowl.
2. Whisk until smooth.
3. Stir in parsley, cilantro, and garlic.
4. Add salt and black pepper to taste.

15. Dips and Spreads

Wholesome and versatile — perfect for dipping, layering, or spreading. Each recipe brings creamy texture and balanced, plant-based flavor.

This section brings together simple, plant-based dips and spreads that work as snacks, appetizers, bowl toppers, or quick additions to everyday meals. Each recipe blends beans, vegetables, herbs, and aromatics into smooth, flavorful mixtures with balanced texture and clean ingredients. Whether you want a classic hummus, a smoky bean dip, a bright veggie spread, or a creamy herb option, these dips are designed to be versatile—perfect for layering on sandwiches, pairing with vegetables, or serving alongside warm pita or crackers.

- Classic Hummus (Base)
- Roasted Red Pepper Hummus
- Smoky Black Bean Dip
- Creamy Spinach and Artichoke Dip
- Edamame Ginger Spread
- Creamy Dill Dip

Classic Hummus (Base)

Smooth, creamy, and endlessly customizable — a true staple for any vegan kitchen.

Makes About 2 cups | Prep Time 10 minutes

Ingredients

1 can (15 ounces) chickpeas, drained and rinsed, or 1½ cups cooked chickpeas

¼ cup fresh lemon juice (about 1 large lemon)

¼ cup tahini

1 garlic clove

2 tablespoons olive oil

½ teaspoon salt

¼ teaspoon cumin

2–4 tablespoons water, as needed for consistency

Directions

Blend chickpeas, lemon juice, tahini, garlic, olive oil, salt, and cumin until smooth. Add water gradually until creamy and fluffy. Adjust seasoning to taste.

Make It Yours Ideas

Swap chickpeas for white beans for a lighter texture.

Add smoked paprika or cayenne for warmth.

Pairs With

Pita, raw vegetables, wraps or grain bowls.

Roasted Red Pepper Hummus

Sweet and smoky with roasted pepper flavor — this twist on classic hummus adds both color and depth.

Makes About 2 cups | Prep Time 10 minutes | Cook Time 25 minutes

Ingredients

1 large red bell pepper, halved and seeded

1 can (15 ounces) chickpeas, drained and rinsed

¼ cup tahini

2 tablespoons olive oil

1 garlic clove

1 tablespoon lemon juice

½ teaspoon smoked paprika

½ teaspoon salt

2–4 tablespoons water, as needed

Directions

1. Preheat oven to 425°F. Roast bell pepper on a parchment-lined sheet, skin side up, until blackened (20–25 minutes).
2. Place in a covered bowl to steam 10 minutes, then peel.
3. Blend roasted pepper with remaining ingredients until smooth, thinning with water to desired texture.

Make It Yours Ideas

Add a spoonful of tomato paste for richness.

Stir in chili flakes or harissa paste.

Pairs With - Flatbreads, sandwiches, or as a dip for roasted vegetables.

Smoky Black Bean Dip

Hearty and flavorful, this protein-packed dip is perfect for tacos, nachos, or spreading on wraps.

Makes About 2 cups | Prep Time 10 minutes | Cook Time 10 minutes

Ingredients

1 can (15 ounces) black beans, drained and rinsed

1 tablespoon olive oil

1 small onion, diced

1 clove garlic, minced

1 teaspoon smoked paprika

½ teaspoon cumin

½ teaspoon salt

¼ cup water or vegetable broth

Juice of ½ lime

Directions

Heat olive oil in a skillet. Add onion and garlic; sauté 3–4 minutes. Stir in smoked paprika and cumin. Add black beans, salt, and water. Simmer 5 minutes. Blend until smooth but still slightly textured. Stir in lime juice.

Make It Yours Ideas

Add roasted corn or chipotle for more complexity.

Stir in minced jalapeño or cayenne.

Pairs With

Tortilla chips, tacos, or veggie wraps.

Creamy Spinach and Artichoke Dip

Classic comfort made vegan — creamy, tangy and perfect fo meal prep.

Makes About 2 cups | Prep Time 15 minutes | Cook Time 15 minutes

Ingredients

1 tablespoon olive oil

1 small onion, diced

2 cloves garlic, minced

1 cup canned or thawed chopped artichoke hearts

2 cups fresh spinach, chopped

1 cup raw cashews, soaked 30 minutes

¾ cup unsweetened plant milk

1 tablespoon lemon juice

2 tablespoons nutritional yeast

½ teaspoon salt

¼ teaspoon black pepper

Directions

Heat olive oil in a skillet. Sauté onion and garlic 5 minutes. Add artichokes and spinach; cook until wilted.

Blend soaked cashews, plant milk, lemon juice, nutritional yeast, salt, and pepper until smooth. Pour sauce into skillet and cook 5 minutes, stirring until thickened.

Make It Yours Ideas

Sprinkle vegan Parmesan or crushed red pepper before serving.

Stir in ¼ teaspoon cayenne or a few dashes of hot sauce.

Pairs With - Crackers, toasted baguette, or baked potatoes.

Edamame Ginger Spread

Bright, green, and lightly spiced — this protein-rich dip pairs beautifully with sushi rolls or as a sandwich spread.

Makes About 2 cups | Prep Time 10 minutes

Ingredients

1½ cups shelled edamame, cooked and cooled

2 tablespoons lime juice

1 tablespoon sesame oil

1 tablespoon soy sauce or tamari

1 garlic clove

1 teaspoon grated fresh ginger

1 tablespoon maple syrup

¼ teaspoon salt

2–4 tablespoons water, as needed

Directions

Blend edamame, lime juice, sesame oil, soy sauce, garlic, ginger, maple syrup, and salt until smooth, adding water to reach desired consistency.

Make It Yours Ideas

Add avocado for extra creaminess or cilantro for freshness.

Blend in wasabi or chili paste.

Pairs With

Rice bowls, sushi rolls or veggie wraps.

Creamy Dill Dip

This creamy, tangy dill dip is perfect for veggie platters, crackers, chips, roasted potatoes, tofu bites, and grain bowls. It holds its shape and thickens in the fridge, making it ideal for appetizers.

Makes About 1¼ cups | Prep Time 10 minutes | Cook Time None

Ingredients

¾ cup plain unsweetened vegan yogurt

¼ cup vegan mayo *or* ¼ cup blended silken tofu

1 tablespoon lemon juice

1 tablespoon apple cider vinegar

1 small clove garlic, grated

1 teaspoon maple syrup

2–3 tablespoons fresh dill, finely chopped

1 tablespoon dried chives *or* 2 tablespoons fresh

½ teaspoon dried parsley

½ teaspoon garlic powder

½ teaspoon onion powder

¼ teaspoon fine sea salt

Black pepper to taste

1–2 teaspoons pickle brine (optional)

Directions

1. Add the vegan yogurt, vegan mayo, lemon juice, vinegar, and grated garlic and maple syrup to a bowl and mix until smooth.
2. Add the dill, chives, parsley, garlic powder, onion powder, salt, and pepper.
3. Stir until evenly combined.

4. Taste and adjust salt, lemon, or dill. Add pickle brine, if desired.
5. Refrigerate for 20–30 minutes before serving.

Make It Yours Ideas

Add chopped pickles for a dill-pickle dip.

Add 1 tbsp (15 mL) olive oil for extra richness.

Add a pinch of smoked paprika for warmth.

Serving Ideas

Serve with raw veggies, crackers, pretzels, or chips.

Use as a spread for wraps and sandwiches.

Dollop on baked potatoes or bowl recipes.

Use as a dip for tofu bites or chickpea fritters.

16. Non-Dairy Yogurts and Cheeses

Creamy, tangy, and full of life — these plant-based yogurts and cheeses prove that comfort food doesn't need compromise.

Each recipe starts with simple ingredients and ends with richness and balance: cashews and coconuts for silkiness, almonds for lightness, tofu for structure, and a sprinkle of nutritional yeast for depth. Whether you're layering tofu ricotta into lasagna, topping pasta with cashew Parmesan, or spooning creamy yogurt over fruit, these recipes bring the familiar flavors you love into a plantsy, homemade form that feels both nourishing and natural.

- Coconut Yogurt (Base)
- Almond Yogurt
- Cashew Yogurt
- Simple Tofu 'Ricotta'
- Cashew 'Parmesan'

Coconut Yogurt (Base)

Thick, creamy, and subtly tangy — a perfect foundation for breakfast bowls, parfaits, or savory dips.

Makes About 2 cups | Prep Time 10 minutes | Ferment time: 12–24 hours

Ingredients

1 can (13.5 ounces) full-fat coconut milk

2 teaspoons cornstarch or tapioca starch

1 teaspoon maple syrup or agave

2 vegan probiotic capsules (use powder only)

Directions

1. Whisk coconut milk and cornstarch in a small saucepan. Warm over medium heat, stirring constantly, until slightly thickened — about 5 minutes.
2. Remove from heat and cool to lukewarm.
3. Stir in maple syrup and probiotic powder.
4. Pour into a clean glass jar, cover loosely with a cloth, and let sit at room temperature 12–24 hours until tangy.
5. Refrigerate to thicken before serving.

Make It Yours Ideas

Add vanilla extract or shredded coconut for a breakfast-style yogurt.

Stir in grated ginger or cinnamon for a warming twist.

Pairs With

Granola, fruit, savory sauces, or smoothies.

Almond Yogurt

Light and nutty with a subtle tang — a great alternative for those who prefer a milder flavor.

Makes About 2 cups | Prep Time 15 minutes | Ferment time: 12–24 hours

Ingredients

1 cup raw almonds, soaked 8 hours and drained

1 ½ cups filtered water

1 tablespoon maple syrup

2 vegan probiotic capsules (use powder only)

Directions

1. Blend soaked almonds and water on high until smooth. Strain through a nut-milk bag for a fine texture. Pour into a saucepan and warm gently 5 minutes over low heat.
2. Cool to lukewarm, stir in maple syrup and probiotic powder, then transfer to a clean jar.
3. Cover loosely and ferment 12–24 hours at room temperature. Refrigerate before serving.

Make It Yours Ideas

Add ½ teaspoon vanilla or a spoonful of lemon juice for brightness.

Stir in cardamom or nutmeg for a dessert-style version.

Pairs With

Oat bowls, fruit compotes, or as a base for creamy dressings.

Cashew Yogurt

Velvety smooth and naturally rich — this yogurt doubles beautifully as a creamy topping or savory dip.

Makes About 2 cups | Prep Time 10 minutes | Ferment time: 12–24 hours

Ingredients

1 cup raw cashews, soaked 4–6 hours

¾ cup filtered water

1 tablespoon lemon juice

2 teaspoons maple syrup

2 vegan probiotic capsules (use powder only)

Directions

Blend soaked cashews, water, lemon juice, and maple syrup until completely smooth. Transfer to a clean glass jar and stir in probiotic powder. Cover loosely with a cloth and let ferment 12–24 hours at room temperature, until tangy and thickened. Chill before using.

Make It Yours Ideas

Blend in a few berries or mango for a fruit-style yogurt.

Add a pinch of turmeric and cumin for a savory version to use in sauces.

Pairs With

Parfaits, sauces, baked potatoes, or savory bowls.

Simple Tofu 'Ricotta'

Soft, spreadable, and lightly seasoned — a perfect replacement for traditional ricotta in pasta, lasagna, or sandwiches.

Makes About 2 cups | Prep Time 10 minutes

Ingredients

1 package (14 ounces) firm tofu, drained

2 tablespoons lemon juice

1 tablespoon olive oil

1 tablespoon nutritional yeast

1 teaspoon apple cider vinegar

½ teaspoon salt

¼ teaspoon garlic powder

¼ teaspoon black pepper

Directions

Crumble tofu into a bowl. Add remaining ingredients and mash with a fork or pulse in a food processor until slightly creamy but still textured.

Make It Yours Ideas

Add fresh basil or parsley for a herbed version.

Mix in crushed red pepper or a touch of smoked paprika.

Pairs With

Lasagna, stuffed shells, toast or wraps.

Cashew 'Parmesan'

Savory, salty, and perfectly crumbly — a quick shake of this on top instantly finishes a dish.

Makes About 2 cups | Prep Time 5 minutes

Ingredients

1 cup raw cashews

¼ cup nutritional yeast

1 teaspoon garlic powder

½ teaspoon salt

Directions

Pulse all ingredients in a food processor until a fine, crumbly texture forms. Store in a sealed jar in the refrigerator for up to 3 weeks.

Make It Yours Ideas

Add ½ teaspoon lemon zest for brightness.

Add ¼ teaspoon smoked paprika for depth.

Stir in crushed chili flakes for a "spicy Parm."

Pairs With

Pasta, grain bowls, soups, or roasted vegetables.

17. Flavor-Enhancing Add-Ons

Quick, versatile enhancements — drizzles, spreads, and infusions that elevate any dish from simple to signature.

This section features small but impactful additions that instantly lift the flavor of any dish. These drizzles, spreads, and infused oils are simple to prepare and designed to complement a wide range of meals—from bowls and salads to roasted vegetables, tofu, and grain dishes. Whether you need a bright citrus finish, a velvety cream-style drizzle, a rich reduction, or a quick herb infusion, these recipes add depth, balance, and a signature touch without extra effort.

- Cashew 'La Crema' Sauce
- Coconut Lime Drizzle
- Balsamic Reduction
- Maple Miso Butter
- Garlic Confit
- Lemon Herb Oil
- Simple Parsley Herb Sauce

Cashew 'La Crema' Sauce

Light, silky, and endlessly versatile — this cream-style base adds body to pastas, soups, or roasted vegetables.

Makes About 2 cups | Prep Time 10 minutes | Soak time: 30 minutes

Ingredients

1 cup raw cashews, soaked 30 minutes

¾ cup warm water

1 tablespoon lemon juice

1 tablespoon olive oil

½ teaspoon salt

¼ teaspoon black pepper

Directions

Blend soaked cashews, water, lemon juice, olive oil, salt, and pepper until perfectly smooth. Warm gently in a saucepan for 3–5 minutes, stirring constantly.

Make It Yours Ideas

Add 1 tablespoon nutritional yeast for extra creaminess.

Add a splash of apple-cider vinegar for extra tang.

Blend in roasted garlic or a pinch of smoked paprika.

Pairs With

Soups, pasta, tacos or grilled vegetables.

Coconut Lime Drizzle

Tropical, bright, and creamy — a quick sauce that brings freshness to spicy or roasted dishes.

Makes About 2 cups | Prep Time 5 minutes | Cook Time 5 minutes

Ingredients

1 cup canned coconut milk (full-fat)

2 tablespoons lime juice

1 tablespoon maple syrup

1 tablespoon olive oil

½ teaspoon salt

Zest of 1 lime

Directions

Combine all ingredients in a small saucepan. Warm gently for 5 minutes, whisking until slightly thickened and glossy.

Make It Yours Ideas

Add a pinch of shredded coconut for texture.

Include minced chili or a few drops of sriracha.

Pairs With

Rice bowls, grilled tofu, or roasted sweet potatoes.

Balsamic Reduction

A concentrated, syrupy drizzle that instantly elevates roasted vegetables, salads, and grain bowls.

Makes About 2 cups (reduces to ~1 cup after simmering) | Prep Time 5 minutes | Cook Time 20 minutes

Ingredients

2 cups balsamic vinegar

2 tablespoons maple syrup or brown sugar (optional, for sweetness)

Directions

Pour balsamic vinegar into a small saucepan. Add maple syrup if using. Bring to a gentle boil over medium heat, then reduce to a low simmer. Cook 15–20 minutes, stirring occasionally, until thickened enough to coat the back of a spoon. Cool before using.

Make It Yours Ideas

Infuse with a crushed garlic clove or a few sprigs of thyme during simmering, then strain before cooling.

Add a pinch of black pepper or a touch of chili flakes for warmth.

Pairs With

Roasted Brussels sprouts, strawberries, arugula salads or flatbreads.

Maple Miso Butter

Savory-sweet and deeply flavorful, this plant-based "butter" adds instant richness to veggies, grains, or baked tofu.

Makes About 2 cups | Prep Time 10 minutes | Cook Time 5 minutes

Ingredients

½ cup softened vegan butter or coconut oil

2 tablespoons white miso paste

1 tablespoon maple syrup

1 tablespoon rice vinegar

½ teaspoon grated ginger

¼ teaspoon black pepper

Directions

Whisk all ingredients together in a bowl until smooth. Warm gently for 2–3 minutes to blend flavors, then cool slightly.

Make It Yours Ideas

Add a splash of sesame oil for nutty aroma.

Stir in chili flakes or a touch of wasabi paste.

Pairs With

Grilled mushrooms, steamed greens, roasted carrots, or noodles.

Garlic Confit

Slow-cooked garlic in oil becomes buttery, mellow, and sweet — a flavor base that keeps beautifully in the fridge.

Makes About 1½ cups | Prep Time 10 minutes | Cook Time 35 minutes

Ingredients

2 heads garlic, cloves peeled

1 cup olive oil (enough to cover cloves)

1 sprig fresh thyme or rosemary (optional)

Directions

1. Place garlic cloves in a small oven-safe dish. Cover completely with olive oil and add herbs if using.
2. Bake at 250°F for 35–40 minutes, until cloves are golden and tender.
3. Cool and store garlic and oil together in a jar in the refrigerator up to 2 weeks.

Make It Yours Ideas

Add a strip of lemon zest for brightness.

Include a pinch of chili flakes while roasting.

Pairs With

Bread, mashed potatoes, pasta sauces, or spreads.

Lemon Herb Oil

Fresh and aromatic — this infused oil adds brightness and a hint of acidity wherever you drizzle it.

Makes About 2 cups | Prep Time 10 minutes | Infuse time: 30 minutes

Ingredients

1 ½ cups olive oil

Zest of 1 large lemon

1 sprig fresh rosemary

3 sprigs fresh thyme

¼ teaspoon salt

Directions

Warm olive oil, lemon zest, rosemary, thyme, and salt in a small saucepan over low heat for 5 minutes. Remove from heat and let steep 30 minutes. Strain and store in a glass jar.

Make It Yours Ideas

Add 1 garlic clove or swap lemon zest for orange.

Infuse with peppercorns or a small, dried chili.

Pairs With

Grain bowls, salads, roasted vegetables, or flatbreads.

Simple Parsley Herb Sauce

A bright green sauce made from fresh herbs, ideal for bowls, potatoes, roasted vegetables, and tofu dishes.

Makes about ¾ cup | Prep Time 10 minutes | Cook Time None

Ingredients

1 cup loosely packed parsley

¼ cup olive oil

2 tablespoons lemon juice

1 small clove garlic

2 tablespoons water

Salt and black pepper to taste

Directions

1. Add all ingredients to a blender or food processor.
2. Blend until smooth.
3. Taste and add more lemon or salt as desired.

18. Drizzles

Quick, flavorful toppings to finish bowls, roasted veggies, or grain dishes with a flourish of color and taste.

Sometimes all a dish needs is a final drizzle to bring it to life. These bright, balanced finishers — from chili-lime oil to balsamic swirl — add color, shine, and that extra bit of magic to your bowl or plate.

- Chili Lime Oil
- Tahini Drizzle
- Balsamic Swirl
- Sweet and Spicy Maple Glaze

Chili Lime Oil

Zesty, spicy, and fragrant — this drizzle adds a punch of brightness and gentle heat.

Makes About 2 cups | Prep Time 5 minutes Cook Time 10 minutes

Ingredients

1 ½ cups olive oil

Zest of 1 lime

Juice of 1 lime (about 2 tablespoons)

2 cloves garlic, smashed

2 teaspoons red pepper flakes (adjust to taste)

½ teaspoon salt

Directions

Warm olive oil in a small saucepan over low heat. Add lime zest, garlic, and red pepper flakes. Cook 5–7 minutes until fragrant but not browned. Remove from heat, stir in lime juice and salt, and let steep 10 minutes. Strain before storing.

Make It Yours Ideas

Add chopped cilantro or a pinch of cumin for depth.

Mix in minced fresh chili for more intensity.

Pairs With

Rice bowls, grilled tofu, roasted cauliflower or tacos.

Tahini Drizzle

Smooth and nutty, this simple sauce transforms vegetables, wraps, or grain bowls into craveable meals.

Makes About 2 cups | Prep Time 10 minutes

Ingredients

½ cup tahini

¼ cup lemon juice

1 tablespoon maple syrup

1 garlic clove, minced

½ teaspoon salt

½ cup warm water (more as needed for consistency)

Directions

Whisk tahini, lemon juice, maple syrup, garlic, and salt together until thick. Slowly whisk in water until smooth and pourable. Adjust thickness to taste.

Make It Yours Ideas

Add 1 teaspoon soy sauce for umami or a pinch of cumin.

Blend in harissa or a small dash of cayenne.

Pairs With

Falafel, roasted veggies, Buddha bowls, or wraps.

Balsamic Swirl

Sweet, tangy, and glossy — a drizzle that gives salads, flatbreads, and roasted vegetables a touch of elegance.

Makes About 1½ cups | Prep Time 5 minutes | Cook Time 15 minutes

Ingredients

2 cups balsamic vinegar

2 tablespoons maple syrup (optional for sweetness)

Directions

Bring balsamic vinegar and maple syrup to a gentle simmer in a small saucepan. Cook 10–15 minutes until reduced by half and syrupy. Cool completely before use.

Make It Yours Ideas

Infuse with a sprig of rosemary or a garlic clove for a savory note.

Add a pinch of black pepper or chili flakes while simmering.

Pairs With

Caprese-style salads, roasted Brussels sprouts or pizza.

Sweet and Spicy Maple Glaze

Sticky, balanced, and bold — this glaze is perfect for coating roasted vegetables, tofu, or tempeh.

Makes About 2 cups | Prep Time 5 minutes | Cook Time 8 minutes

Ingredients

½ cup maple syrup

¼ cup apple cider vinegar

2 tablespoons soy sauce or tamari

1 teaspoon chili flakes

1 teaspoon smoked paprika

1 clove garlic, grated

1 teaspoon cornstarch mixed with 1 tablespoon water

Directions

Combine maple syrup, vinegar, soy sauce, chili flakes, paprika, and garlic in a saucepan. Bring to a simmer over medium heat. Add cornstarch slurry and whisk until thickened, about 2–3 minutes. Cool slightly before use.

Make It Yours Ideas

Replace vinegar with orange juice for citrus brightness.

Use extra chili flakes or a dash of chipotle powder.

Pairs With

Roasted carrots, tempeh, grilled tofu, or baked squash.

19. Comfort Sauces

These are the essentials that make meals craveable — creamy sauces, zesty dips, and fresh toppings that bring balance and contrast to every bite.

This section gathers the sauces that make meals feel satisfying and complete—creamy blends, bold bean-based dips, and zesty toppings that bring richness, contrast, and depth to every bite. These recipes rely on simple, plant-based ingredients like potatoes, tofu, cashews, beans, herbs, and aromatics to create smooth, flavorful finishes that pair easily with bowls, tacos, vegetables, pasta, or baked potatoes. Whether you're looking for a classic "cheese"-style sauce or something with a smoky, spicy, or citrusy twist, these comfort options are designed to give your meals a flavorful, nourishing boost.

- Potato Based 'Cheese' Sauce
- Silky Tofu Based 'Cheese' Sauce
- Cashew Blender 'Cheese' Sauce
- White Bean 'Cheese' Sauce
- How to Cook Beans from Scratch
- Black Bean Sauce
- Spicy Chipotle-Roasted Garlic Black Bean Sauce
- Cilantro Lime Green Black Bean Sauce
- Cashew Black Bean Queso

Potato Based 'Cheese' Sauce

Creamy, rich, and perfectly pourable — this sauce coats pasta beautifully while staying 100% dairy-free.

Makes About 4 cups | Prep Time 10 minutes | Cook Time 15 minutes

Ingredients

1 ½ cups peeled, cubed potatoes

¾ cup chopped carrots

½ cup raw cashews

¼ cup nutritional yeast

2 tablespoons olive oil or vegan butter

1 tablespoon lemon juice

1 teaspoon Dijon mustard

1 teaspoon salt

½ teaspoon garlic powder

½ teaspoon onion powder

½ cup unsweetened plant milk (add more as needed for consistency)

Directions

Boil potatoes, carrots, and cashews together until soft — about 10 minutes. Drain and transfer to a blender. Add nutritional yeast, olive oil, lemon juice, mustard, salt, garlic powder, onion powder, and plant milk. Blend until smooth and creamy. Warm over low heat before serving, thinning with more milk if desired.

Silky Tofu Based 'Cheese' Sauce

This sauce blends soft tofu with simple seasonings to create a smooth, pourable "cheesy" coating for pasta or vegetables. It's light, protein-rich, and comes together quickly in a blender.

Makes about 2 ½-3 cups | Prep time: 10 minutes | Cook time: 5 minutes

Ingredients

1 (12–14 oz) package silken tofu

½ cup unsweetened plant milk

¼ cup nutritional yeast

2 tablespoons avocado oil or olive oil

1 tablespoon lemon juice

1 teaspoon Dijon mustard

1 teaspoon garlic powder

½ teaspoon onion powder

½ teaspoon salt, plus more to taste

¼ teaspoon turmeric (for color)

1–2 teaspoons miso paste or 1 teaspoon soy sauce (optional depth)

Directions

Blend all ingredients until completely smooth. Warm gently in a saucepan for 3–5 minutes until thickened. Taste and adjust salt, brightness, and depth. Toss with 16 ounces cooked macaroni.

Cashew Blender 'Cheese' Sauce

Cashews make a naturally creamy base that turns velvety once blended with warm spices and a touch of nutritional yeast. It delivers a rich, classic-style cheese sauce without much cooking required.

Makes about 2 ½-3 cups | Prep time: 10 minutes | Cook time: 5 minutes

Ingredients

1 cup raw cashews, soaked 15 minutes in hot water

1 cup water or unsweetened plant milk

¼ cup nutritional yeast

2 tablespoons lemon juice

1 tablespoon avocado oil or olive oil

1 teaspoon garlic powder

½ teaspoon onion powder

½ teaspoon smoked paprika or sweet paprika

½ teaspoon salt

1–2 teaspoons tapioca starch (optional for stretchiness)

Directions

Drain the cashews. Blend everything until very smooth. If using tapioca starch, pour sauce into a saucepan and cook 2–3 minutes until it thickens and gets slightly stretchy. Toss with 16 ounces cooked macaroni.

White Bean 'Cheese' Sauce

White beans create a hearty, ultra-smooth sauce with a mild flavor that takes on seasonings beautifully. It's an easy, fiber-packed option that blends into a thick, satisfying "cheesy" coating for pasta.

Makes about 2 ½-3 cups | Prep time: 10 minutes | Cook time: 5 minutes

Ingredients

1½ cups (about 1 can drained) white beans

¾ cup unsweetened plant milk

¼ cup nutritional yeast

2 tablespoons olive oil

2 tablespoons tahini or cashew butter

1 tablespoon lemon juice

1 teaspoon garlic powder

½ teaspoon onion powder

½ teaspoon salt

½ teaspoon smoked paprika or chili powder (optional)

Directions

Blend all ingredients until smooth. Warm 3–5 minutes in a saucepan to thicken slightly. Adjust salt or acidity. Toss with 16 ounces cooked macaroni.

Make It Yours Ideas

Stir in a pinch of smoked paprika or a dash of turmeric for color and warmth. Add a spoonful of chipotle paste or hot sauce for a smoky kick.

Pairs With

Elbow macaroni, steamed broccoli, or roasted cauliflower.

How to Cook Beans from Scratch

A guide for tender, flavorful beans you can use in any sauce, dip, or meal. Works with black beans, pinto, navy, cannellini, chickpeas, or kidney beans.

Makes: About 4–5 cups cooked beans (from 1 cup dry) | Prep Time: 5 minutes | Cook Time: Varies by method

Ingredients

1 cup dry beans, rinsed and sorted

4–6 cups water

1 bay leaf (optional)

1–2 garlic cloves, smashed (optional)

Salt added after cooking (optional)

Stovetop Method

1. Place rinsed beans in a large pot and cover with 4–6 cups of water.
2. Add bay leaf and garlic if using.
3. Bring to a boil over high heat.
4. Reduce heat to low, cover with the lid slightly ajar, and simmer until tender.
5. Check the water level periodically and add more if the beans become exposed.
6. Begin checking for doneness at 45 minutes; some beans may take 90 minutes or longer depending on variety and age.
7. Remove bay leaf and garlic.
8. Drain the beans or keep some cooking liquid for creamier sauces.
9. Season with salt at the end.

Slow Cooker Method

1. Place rinsed beans in a slow cooker and cover with 5–6 cups water.
2. Add bay leaf and garlic if using.
3. Cover and cook on Low for 6–8 hours or High for 3–4 hours, until tender.
4. Remove bay leaf and garlic.
5. Drain or keep cooking liquid as desired.
6. Season with salt at the end.

Quick-Soak Method (Optional)

1. Place rinsed beans in a large pot and cover with water by 2–3 inches.
2. Bring to a full boil and boil for 2 minutes.
3. Turn off heat, cover, and let sit for 1 hour.
4. Drain and rinse beans.
5. Proceed with the stovetop method, reducing simmer time by 20–25%.

No-Soak Stovetop Method

1. Place rinsed beans in a large pot and cover with 5–6 cups water.
2. Add bay leaf or garlic if desired.
3. Bring to a boil over high heat.
4. Reduce heat to low, cover, and simmer until beans are tender.
5. Check water level periodically and add more as needed.
6. Expect longer cook times; some varieties may take 2 hours or more.
7. Remove bay leaf and garlic.
8. Drain or reserve cooking liquid.
9. Season with salt at the end.

Why Salt Is Added After Cooking

Salt can slow the softening of bean skins as they cook. Adding it early may keep beans firm even after long simmering. Seasoning at the end ensures the beans soften fully and absorb flavor more evenly.

Approximate Cooking Times by Variety

Black Beans: 60–75 minutes stovetop (soaked); 90+ minutes no-soak; 6–7 hours slow cooker

Pinto Beans: 75–90 minutes stovetop; 2 hours no-soak; 7–8 hours slow cooker

Chickpeas: 90+ minutes stovetop; 2–3 hours no-soak; 8+ hours slow cooker

Kidney Beans: 90 minutes stovetop; 2 hours no-soak; 7–8 hours slow cooker

Navy/Cannellini Beans: 60–75 minutes stovetop; 90+ minutes no-soak; 6–7 hours slow cooker

Notes

For *creamier* bean sauces, keep up to 1 cup of the cooking liquid.

For *firmer* beans, drain fully and rinse.

For *extra flavor*, add a small piece of onion, a celery rib, or a teaspoon of dried herbs to the pot.

Important Note About Kidney Beans

Kidney beans must be boiled before simmering or slow cooking. Undercooked kidney beans contain a naturally occurring compound (phytohaemagglutinin) that can cause digestive illness. Always bring kidney beans to a full boil for at least 10 minutes before reducing to a simmer. Do not cook dry kidney beans in a slow cooker without boiling them first.

Black Bean Sauce

Creamy, savory, and rich, this sauce delivers depth similar to queso or enchilada-style toppings. It blends smoothly, reheats well, and works across bowls, tacos, nachos, vegetables, and more.

Makes about 1¾ cups | Prep time: 10 minutes | Cook time: 10 minutes

Ingredients

1 tablespoon olive oil

½ cup diced onion

2 cloves garlic, minced

1 can (15 ounces) black beans, drained and rinsed

½ cup vegetable broth

2 tablespoons lime juice

1 tablespoon tomato paste

1 teaspoon ground cumin

½ teaspoon smoked paprika

¼ teaspoon chili powder

¼ teaspoon fine sea salt, plus more to taste

Black pepper to taste

1 tablespoon tahini OR cashew butter (adds creaminess and depth)

1 tablespoon nutritional yeast (adds mild cheesy richness)

Pinch of cayenne or a few slices jalapeño (adds balanced heat)

Directions

1. Warm the olive oil in a saucepan over medium heat and add the onion. Cook until softened.
2. Add the garlic and cook for 1 minute.

3. Add the black beans, vegetable broth, lime juice, tomato paste, cumin, smoked paprika, chili powder, salt, black pepper, tahini or cashew butter, nutritional yeast, and cayenne or jalapeño. Stir to combine.
4. Simmer for 5–7 minutes to allow the flavors to blend.
5. Transfer the mixture to a blender and blend until smooth.
6. Return the sauce to the saucepan if needed to warm through and adjust seasoning.

Serving Ideas

Drizzle over a baked or air-fried sweet potato.

Use as a nacho sauce over tortilla chips with roasted corn, salsa, and avocado.

Spoon into taco bowls with quinoa, veggies, and shredded lettuce.

Add as a layer inside enchiladas before rolling.

Use as a dip for roasted vegetables or sweet potato wedges.

Spicy Chipotle–Roasted Garlic Black Bean Sauce

Deep, smoky, and spicy, this sauce layers chipotle heat with mellow roasted garlic. Ideal for nachos, burrito bowls, tacos, and roasted sweet potatoes.

Makes About 1¾ cups | Prep Time 10 minutes | Cook Time 20 minutes

Ingredients

1 tablespoon olive oil

1 small head garlic

½ cup diced onion

1 can (15 ounces) black beans, drained and rinsed

½ cup vegetable broth

1 tablespoon lime juice

1 tablespoon tomato paste

1–2 teaspoons adobo sauce, from canned chipotles

½ teaspoon ground cumin

½ teaspoon smoked paprika

¼ teaspoon chili powder

¼ teaspoon fine sea salt

Black pepper, to taste

1 tablespoon tahini *or* cashew butter

Splash of vinegar (optional)

Directions

1. Preheat the oven to 400°F. Slice the top off the garlic head, drizzle lightly with olive oil, wrap in foil, and roast until soft.
2. Warm the olive oil in a saucepan over medium heat and add the onion. Cook until softened. Add the roasted garlic cloves, black beans, vegetable broth, lime juice, tomato paste, adobo sauce, cumin, smoked paprika, chili powder, salt, and black pepper. Stir to combine.
3. Simmer for 5–7 minutes. Blend the mixture until smooth. Add tahini or cashew butter and blend again until creamy.
4. Return to the pan to warm if needed and adjust seasoning. Add a splash of vinegar, if desired, for extra brightness.

Cilantro Lime Green Black Bean Sauce

Fresh, herbal, and bright, this version blends cilantro and extra lime to create a green-tinted bean sauce perfect for bowls, nachos, or spooned over roasted sweet potatoes.

Makes About 1¾ cups | Prep Time 10 minutes | Cook Time 10 minutes

Ingredients

1 tablespoon olive oil
½ cup diced onion
2 cloves garlic, minced
1 can (15 ounces) black beans, drained and rinsed
½ cup vegetable broth
3 tablespoons lime juice
1 tablespoon tomato paste
½ teaspoon cumin
¼ teaspoon smoked paprika
¼ teaspoon fine sea salt
Black pepper to taste
Zest of 1 organic lime
1 tablespoon cashew butter
¼ cup fresh cilantro leaves, packed

Directions

1. Warm the olive oil in a saucepan over medium heat and add the onion. Cook until softened. Add the garlic and cook for 1 minute.
2. Add the black beans, vegetable broth, lime juice, tomato paste, cumin, smoked paprika, salt, and black pepper.
3. Simmer for 5 minutes.
4. Blend the mixture with cilantro until smooth. Add cashew butter and blend again. Return to the pan to warm, add fresh lime zest and adjust seasoning.

Make It Yours Ideas - Add jalapeño or serrano for a spicy green version.

Add avocado for extra creaminess (blend and serve immediately).

Cashew Black Bean Queso

Creamy, rich, and queso-inspired, this variation blends soaked cashews with black beans and spices for a dip-style sauce that works with nachos, bowls, quesadillas, roasted veggies, and sweet potatoes.

Makes About 2 cups | Prep Time 10 minutes | Cook Time 10 minutes

Ingredients

½ cup raw cashews, soaked in hot water for 15 minutes

1 tablespoon olive oil

½ cup diced onion

2 cloves garlic, minced

1 can (15 ounces) black beans, drained and rinsed

½ cup vegetable broth

1 tablespoon lime juice

1 tablespoon tomato paste

2 tablespoons nutritional yeast

½ teaspoon cumin

½ teaspoon smoked paprika

¼ teaspoon chili powder

¼ teaspoon fine sea salt

Black pepper to taste

Optional Extras

1–2 tablespoons pickled jalapeño brine for tang

Pinch of turmeric for color

Roasted red pepper for a smoky, slightly sweet finish

Directions

1. Drain the cashews.
2. Warm the olive oil in a saucepan over medium heat and add the onion. Cook until softened.
3. Add the garlic and cook for 1 minute.
4. Add the black beans, vegetable broth, lime juice, tomato paste, nutritional yeast, cumin, smoked paprika, chili powder, salt, and black pepper. Stir to combine.
5. Simmer for 5 minutes.
6. Blend the mixture with the soaked cashews until completely smooth.
7. Return to the saucepan, warm gently, and adjust seasoning.

20. Fresh Classics

This section highlights vibrant, ready-to-serve sauces and toppings made with fresh herbs, citrus, aromatics, and vegetables. Each recipe delivers clean, lively flavor that comes together quickly—perfect for spooning over bowls, tacos, grain dishes, salads, or roasted vegetables. From creamy dill blends to bright salsas, guacamole, and herby sauces, these fresh classics bring lift, contrast, and balance to everyday meals with minimal preparation and dependable results.

- Classic Guacamole
- Mild Fresh Salsa
- Spicy Salsa Roja
- Green Tomatillo Salsa (Salsa Verde)
- Mock 'Sour Cream'
- Chimichurri Sauce
- Lemon Dill Tahini Sauce
- Greek Style Dill Sauce (Vegan Tzatziki)
- Dill Avocado Green Sauce

Classic Guacamole

Creamy, balanced, and fresh — the perfect topping for tacos, bowls, or toast.

Makes About 2 cups | Prep Time 10 minutes

Ingredients

3 ripe avocados

1 small tomato, diced

¼ cup finely chopped red onion

2 tablespoons chopped cilantro

1 tablespoon lime juice

½ teaspoon salt

¼ teaspoon black pepper

Directions

Mash avocados in a bowl until mostly smooth. Stir in tomato, onion, cilantro, lime juice, salt, and pepper. Adjust lime and salt to taste.

Make It Yours Ideas

Add diced mango or corn for a sweet variation.

Mix in minced jalapeño or chili flakes.

Pairs With

Tacos, grain bowls, burritos or avocado toast.

Mild Fresh Salsa

Bright, juicy, and balanced — a simple table salsa that keeps the focus on freshness.

Makes About 2 cups | Prep Time 10 minutes

Ingredients

3 medium tomatoes, finely diced

¼ cup finely chopped red onion

2 tablespoons chopped cilantro

1 tablespoon lime juice

½ teaspoon salt

¼ teaspoon black pepper

Directions

Combine all ingredients in a bowl and stir gently. Let sit 15 minutes before serving to allow flavors to blend.

Make It Yours Ideas

Add diced cucumber or mango for extra freshness.

Include a small pinch of cayenne or chili powder.

Pairs With

Tacos, salads, grain bowls, or as a dip for chips.

Spicy Salsa Roja

Bold, smoky and rich — ideal for tacos, roasted vegetables, or as a base for enchilada sauce.

Makes About 2 cups | Prep Time 10 minutes | Cook Time 15 minutes

Ingredients

4 medium tomatoes, halved

2 cloves garlic, unpeeled

1 small jalapeño or serrano pepper

¼ small onion, peeled

1 tablespoon olive oil

1 tablespoon lime juice

½ teaspoon salt

Directions

Broil tomatoes, garlic, pepper, and onion on a lined baking sheet until lightly charred, about 8–10 minutes. Peel garlic, then transfer everything to a blender with olive oil, lime juice, and salt. Blend until smooth.

Make It Yours Ideas

Use roasted tomatillos instead of tomatoes for a tangy twist.

Add an extra pepper or a pinch of chipotle powder.

Pairs With

Burrito bowls, roasted potatoes, or tacos.

Green Tomatillo Salsa (Salsa Verde)

A bright, tangy sauce made from fresh tomatillos. Tomatillos come wrapped in a papery husk, and once removed, their surface feels slightly sticky — this is natural and rinses off easily. You can enjoy them raw for a sharper flavor or simmer them briefly for a softer, more blended sauce. This salsa works well as a topping for bowls, tacos, roasted vegetables, beans, or as a dip with chips.

Makes about 1½ cups | Prep Time 10 minutes | Cook Time 5 minutes (optional)

Ingredients

6–7 medium tomatillos (about 12 ounces), husks removed

1 small jalapeño or serrano pepper, stem removed

1 clove garlic

½ small white onion, chopped

¼ cup chopped cilantro

Juice of ½ lime

Salt to taste

Directions

1. Remove the papery husks from the tomatillos.
2. Rinse the tomatillos under warm water until the natural sticky coating is gone.
3. Chop the tomatillos into quarters if using raw.
4. For a softer, mellower salsa, place the tomatillos and jalapeño in a small saucepan, cover with water, and simmer 5 minutes.
5. Drain the tomatillos and jalapeño, if simmered.
6. Add the tomatillos, jalapeño, garlic, onion, and cilantro to a blender or food processor.
7. Add the lime juice and salt.

8. Blend the mixture until smooth or pulse for a chunkier texture.
9. Taste the salsa and adjust salt or lime as desired.

Uses

Spoon over grain bowls, roasted vegetables, burritos, tacos, or tofu scrambles.

Stir into rice or quinoa for extra brightness.

Use as a quick simmer sauce for beans or roasted chickpeas.

Serve as a chip dip or drizzle over salads or baked potatoes.

Roasted Tomatillo Salsa

For a deeper, slightly smoky flavor, roast the tomatillos, jalapeño, and onion at 425°F until lightly charred, then blend with the remaining ingredients. The roasting concentrates the tomatillos' natural tartness and adds a richer body to the sauce.

Avocado Tomatillo Salsa

Blend the finished salsa with half of a ripe avocado for a creamier texture and a softer tang. This variation works especially well as a topping for bowls, tacos, wraps, and grilled vegetables.

Smoky Salsa Verde

Add a pinch of smoked paprika or a small roasted poblano pepper to the blender. This creates a slightly smoky finish that pairs beautifully with roasted potatoes, beans, and tofu.

Cilantro Lime Salsa Verde

Increase the cilantro and add the juice of an additional ½ lime for a brighter, more herby version. This is excellent as a dressing for salads, grain bowls, and roasted chickpeas.

Spicy Salsa Verde

Leave the seeds in the jalapeño or swap it for a serrano or small green chile. The extra heat balances the natural acidity and creates a lively kick that works well with tacos, nachos, and vegetable skewers.

Mock Sour 'Cream'

Smooth and tangy— the essential cool contrast for spicy dishes.

Makes About 2 cups | Prep Time 10 minutes | Soak time: 30 minutes

Ingredients

1 cup raw cashews, soaked 30 minutes

¾ cup water

1 tablespoon lemon juice

1 tablespoon apple cider vinegar

½ teaspoon salt

Directions

Blend soaked cashews, water, lemon juice, vinegar, and salt until perfectly smooth. Chill before serving.

Make It Yours Ideas

Add a spoonful of vegan yogurt for extra tang.

Stir in chipotle, smoked paprika or chives for variation.

Pairs With

Tacos, baked potatoes, chili, or nachos.

Chimichurri Sauce

A fresh, herbal sauce from Argentina that pairs beautifully with roasted vegetables, tofu, grains, and warm salads.

Makes about ⅔ cup | Prep Time 10 minutes | Cook Time None

Ingredients

1 cup finely chopped fresh parsley

2 tablespoons chopped fresh oregano or ½ teaspoon dried

2 cloves garlic, minced

¼ cup olive oil

2 tablespoons red wine vinegar

1 tablespoon lemon juice

¼ teaspoon crushed red pepper flakes

Salt and black pepper to taste

Directions

1. Add parsley, oregano, and garlic to a bowl.
2. Add olive oil, vinegar, lemon juice, and pepper flakes.
3. Stir the mixture until combined.
4. Add salt and black pepper to taste.

Lemon Dill Tahini Sauce

Creamy, bright, and earthy, this sauce is excellent over bowls, roasted vegetables, chickpea patties, grains, or drizzled on wraps.

Makes About 1 cup | Prep Time 10 minutes | Cook Time None

Ingredients

⅓ cup tahini

3 tablespoons lemon juice

¼ cup water, plus more as needed

1 tablespoon olive oil

1 tablespoon maple syrup

1 small clove garlic, grated

2–3 tablespoons fresh dill, finely chopped

¼ teaspoon fine sea salt

Black pepper to taste

Zest of ½ lemon (optional)

1 tablespoon white wine vinegar for extra tang (optional)

Directions

1. Add the tahini, lemon juice, water, olive oil, maple syrup, and garlic to a bowl and whisk until smooth.
2. Add the fresh dill, salt, and black pepper.
3. Whisk again until creamy. Add additional water to thin if needed.
4. Chill for 20 minutes before using.

Make It Yours Ideas - Add lemon zest for extra brightness.

Add 1 tablespoon vegan yogurt for a softer, tangier finish.

Greek Style Dill Sauce (Vegan Tzatziki)

This vegan tzatziki-style sauce is fresh, creamy, and perfect for bowls, pitas, roasted vegetables, salads, or as a topping for crispy chickpeas or tofu.

Servings: Makes About 1¼ cups | Prep Time 15 minutes | Cook Time None

Ingredients

1 cup plain unsweetened vegan yogurt

½ cup finely grated cucumber, squeezed dry

1 tablespoon lemon juice

1 tablespoon olive oil

1 small clove garlic, grated

2 tablespoon fresh dill, finely chopped

¼ teaspoon fine sea salt

Black pepper to taste

1 tablespoon white wine vinegar

Zest of ½ lemon

2 tablespoons fresh mint, finely chopped

Directions

1. Add the vegan yogurt, grated cucumber, lemon juice, olive oil, garlic, dill, salt, and black pepper to a bowl and stir until smooth.
2. Add the vinegar, lemon zest or chopped mint.
3. Mix again until evenly blended.
4. Chill for 30 minutes to allow flavors to develop.

Dill Avocado Green Sauce

Creamy, vibrant, and naturally green, this sauce pairs well with bowls, roasted vegetables, tacos, salads, or spooned over a sweet potato.

Makes About 1¼ cups | Prep Time 10 minutes | Cook Time None

Ingredients

1 ripe avocado

1 tablespoon vegan yogurt (optional, for creaminess)

¼ cup water

2 tablespoons lemon juice

1 tablespoon olive oil

1 clove garlic

2–3 tablespoons fresh dill, chopped

¼ teaspoon fine sea salt

Black pepper to taste

1 tablespoon white wine vinegar (optional, for brightness)

1 handful fresh parsley or cilantro (optional for color)

Directions

1. Add the avocado, vegan yogurt (if using), water, lemon juice, olive oil, garlic, dill, salt, and pepper to a blender and blend until smooth.
2. Add water if needed to thin. Add parsley or cilantro if using and blend again. Taste and adjust salt or lemon.

Make It Yours Ideas

Add jalapeño for a spicy sauce.

21. Jams and Marmalades

Bright, tangy, and naturally sweet — these fruit spreads bring color and contrast to both savory and sweet plates.

Simple fruit, a touch of sweetness, and a bit of time — that's all it takes to capture the taste of each season. These jams and marmalades are made for more than breakfast; they're designed to layer across your meals, adding brightness, contrast, or a pop of color wherever you need it.

Spoon them over toast or yogurt, pair them with vegan cheese, or brush them onto vegetables before roasting. However, when you use them, they'll remind you that the simplest ingredients often create the most memorable flavors.

- Classic Orange Marmalade
- Strawberry Basil Jam
- Mixed Berry Chia Jam
- Sweet Pepper Jam
- Peach Ginger Jam
- Green Cilantro Chutney
- Cranberry Apple Chutney

Classic Orange Marmalade

Sweet, slightly bitter, and fragrant — the perfect balance of citrus brightness and gentle caramelized depth.

Makes About 2 cups | Prep Time 15 minutes | Cook Time 45 minutes

Ingredients

3 medium oranges (preferably thin-skinned)

1 lemon

2 cups water

1 cup coconut sugar

Directions

Wash oranges and lemon well. Slice thinly, removing seeds. Combine all fruit and water in a saucepan. Simmer for 30 minutes, stirring occasionally, until peels soften. Add sugar and cook 15–20 minutes longer, stirring often, until thickened and glossy. Cool before storing in jars.

Make It Yours Ideas

Use half oranges and half blood oranges for deeper color.

Add a cinnamon stick or a few cloves during cooking, then remove before cooling.

Pairs With

Toast, crepes, vegan cheeses, or as a glaze for roasted carrots or tofu.

Strawberry Basil Jam

Fresh, aromatic, and slightly floral — a spring favorite that doubles as a topping or dessert sauce.

Makes About 2 cups | Prep Time 10 minutes | Cook Time 25 minutes

Ingredients

2 cups chopped fresh strawberries

½ cup coconut sugar

2 tablespoons lemon juice

1 tablespoon finely chopped fresh basil

Directions

Simmer strawberries, sugar, and lemon juice in a saucepan over medium heat until thickened — about 20–25 minutes. Stir in basil and remove from heat. Cool completely before storing.

Make It Yours Ideas

Replace basil with mint or thyme for a different note.

Add a pinch of black pepper or grated ginger.

Pairs With

Toast, yogurt, vegan ice cream, or savory paninis.

Mixed Berry Chia Jam

Quick, nutrient-rich, and no refined sugar — thickened naturally with chia seeds for an easy refrigerator jam.

Makes About 2 cups | Prep Time 5 minutes | Cook Time 10 minutes

Ingredients

2 cups mixed berries (fresh or frozen)

2 tablespoons maple syrup

1 tablespoon lemon juice

2 tablespoons chia seeds

Directions

Simmer berries, maple syrup, and lemon juice over medium heat until berries soften — about 5–7 minutes. Mash lightly, then stir in chia seeds. Cook 2–3 minutes more. Remove from heat. Let thicken as it cools.

Make It Yours Ideas

Swap berries for peaches, cherries, or figs.

Add cinnamon, cardamom, or orange zest.

Pairs With

Toast, overnight oats, parfaits, or peanut butter sandwiches.

Sweet Pepper Jam

Vibrant, glossy, and full of personality — a sweet-heat condiment that pairs perfectly with vegan cheeses and roasted vegetables.

Makes About 2 cups | Prep Time 10 minutes | Cook Time 30 minutes

Ingredients

3 red bell peppers, finely diced

1 small red chili pepper, minced (or ½ teaspoon red pepper flakes)

1 cup coconut sugar

½ cup apple cider vinegar

½ teaspoon salt

Directions

Combine all ingredients in a saucepan. Bring to a simmer and cook 25–30 minutes, stirring often, until mixture thickens and becomes syrupy. Remove from heat and cool completely before storing.

Make It Yours Ideas

Use half red and half orange peppers for a golden hue.

Add an extra chili or a dash of smoked paprika.

Pairs With

Vegan cheese boards, sandwiches, bean burgers, or as a glaze for tofu.

Peach Ginger Jam

Warm, gently spicy, and golden — a perfect late-summer preserve that's as good on toast as in marinades.

Makes About 2 cups | Prep Time 10 minutes | Cook Time 25 minutes

Ingredients

3 cups chopped ripe peaches (peeled)

½ cup coconut sugar

1 tablespoon grated fresh ginger

1 tablespoon lemon juice

Directions

Simmer peaches, sugar, ginger, and lemon juice in a saucepan over medium heat until fruit breaks down and mixture thickens — about 20–25 minutes. Mash lightly for a rustic texture or blend briefly for smooth jam.

Make It Yours Ideas

Mix in a few raspberries for color and tartness.

Add a pinch of cinnamon or nutmeg for a warm flavor.

Pairs With

Oat bowls, crepes, or as a glaze for grilled fruit or tempeh.

Green Cilantro Chutney

A fresh, sharp sauce that pairs well with bowls, roasted vegetables, tofu, and naan-style flatbreads.

Makes about ¾ cup | Prep Time 10 minutes | Cook Time None

Ingredients

1 cup cilantro leaves

¼ cup mint leaves (optional)

1 small clove garlic

1 tablespoon lemon juice

1 tablespoon water

1 tablespoon olive oil

½ teaspoon salt

Pinch of cayenne or black pepper

Directions

1. Add all ingredients to a blender or food processor.
2. Blend until smooth.
3. Taste and adjust lemon or salt.

Cranberry Apple Chutney

Sweet, tangy, and gently spiced — this chutney pairs beautifully with savory dishes and also shines on toast or grain bowls.

Makes About 2 cups | Prep Time 10 minutes | Cook Time 15 minutes

Ingredients

2 cups fresh cranberries

1 medium apple, peeled and finely diced

½ cup water

½ cup coconut sugar or maple syrup

2 tablespoons apple cider vinegar

¼ cup finely chopped onion

¼ teaspoon cinnamon

¼ teaspoon ginger

Pinch of salt

Directions

Combine cranberries, apple, water, coconut sugar, vinegar, onion, cinnamon, ginger, and salt in a saucepan. Bring to a simmer and cook 12–15 minutes, stirring occasionally, until thickened and glossy. Cool before serving.

Make It Yours Ideas

Add raisins or chopped dates for a deeper sweetness.

Add a pinch of chili flakes for sweet heat.

Pairs With

Portabella steaks, grain bowls, roasted sweet potatoes, sandwiches or toast.

22. Dessert Drizzles

Velvety, natural sweetness made from whole ingredients — perfect for topping fruit, oatmeal, pancakes, or desserts.

These sauces prove that sweetness can still be wholesome and intentional. Each recipe starts with real ingredients — nuts, fruit, dates, maple, and spice — blended or simmered into silky drizzles that bring warmth and richness to breakfast, dessert, or snacks. Use them over pancakes, oatmeal, vegan ice cream, or fresh fruit for a touch of indulgence that stays true to clean, simple cooking. They're the kind of staples that make everyday moments feel just a little more special.

- Hazelnut Chocolate Spread
- Salted Caramel Date Sauce
- Maple Ginger Sauce
- Berry Balsamic Drizzle
- Chocolate Sauce
- Salted Chocolate Sauce
- Orange Infused Chocolate Sauce
- Mint Chocolate Sauce
- Mocha Chocolate Sauce
- Spiced Mexican Chocolate Sauce
- Maple Cinnamon Chocolate Sauce
- Coconut Almond Chocolate Sauce

Hazelnut Chocolate Spread

Rich, smooth, and reminiscent of Nutella — but cleaner, simpler, and fully plant-based.

Makes About 2 cups | Prep Time 10 minutes | Cook Time 10 minutes

Ingredients

2 cups roasted hazelnuts

¼ cup cocoa powder

¼ cup maple syrup

½ teaspoon vanilla extract

¼ teaspoon salt

¼ cup warm water (or as needed for blending)

Directions

Blend roasted hazelnuts in a food processor 5–7 minutes until creamy. Add cocoa, maple syrup, vanilla, salt, and water. Blend again until smooth and glossy.

Make It Yours Ideas

Add 1 tablespoon melted coconut oil for extra shine.

Stir in a pinch of cinnamon or espresso powder.

Pairs With

Fruit, toast, oatmeal or layered parfaits.

Salted Caramel Date Sauce

Thick, gooey, and naturally sweetened with dates — no refined sugar needed.

Makes About 2 cups | Prep Time 10 minutes | Cook Time 5 minutes

Ingredients

1 cup pitted Medjool dates

¾ cup warm water

¼ cup coconut milk

1 teaspoon vanilla extract

½ teaspoon sea salt

Directions

Soak dates in warm water for 10 minutes. Blend with remaining ingredients until smooth and creamy. Warm before serving if desired.

Make It Yours Ideas

Add 1 tablespoon nut butter for extra richness.

Stir in a dash of cinnamon.

Pairs With

Apple slices, banana ice cream or coffee drinks.

Maple Ginger Sauce

Warm, aromatic, and silky — drizzle it over pancakes, roasted pears, or ice cream.

Makes About 2 cups | Prep Time 5 minutes | Cook Time 10 minutes

Ingredients

½ cup maple syrup

½ cup coconut milk

1 tablespoon grated fresh ginger

½ teaspoon vanilla extract

Pinch of salt

Directions

Combine all ingredients in a small saucepan. Simmer gently for 8–10 minutes until slightly thickened. Remove from heat and cool.

Make It Yours Ideas

Replace coconut milk with almond milk for a lighter version.

Add a pinch of nutmeg or cardamom.

Pairs With

Pancakes, vegan ice cream or baked fruit.

Berry Balsamic Drizzle

Sweet and tangy, with just a touch of depth from balsamic — perfect for desserts or brunch dishes.

Makes About 2 cups | Prep Time 10 minutes | Cook Time 15 minutes

Ingredients

2 cups mixed berries (fresh or frozen)

2 tablespoons balsamic vinegar

2 tablespoons maple syrup

½ teaspoon vanilla extract

Directions

Simmer berries, vinegar, and maple syrup in a saucepan 10–15 minutes, until thick and syrupy. Remove from heat, stir in vanilla, and strain if desired.

Make It Yours Ideas

Use all strawberries or all blueberries for a single-note flavor.

Add black pepper or a touch of fresh basil.

Pairs With

Waffles, parfaits, vegan yogurt or cheesecake.

Chocolate Sauce

This smooth and versatile chocolate sauce uses pantry staples and creates a pourable consistency that stays silky as it cools. Great for desserts, fruit, waffles, or layering into parfaits.

Makes About 1 cup | Prep Time 5 minutes | Cook Time 5 minutes

Ingredients

½ cup water

⅓ cup unsweetened cocoa powder

½ cup maple syrup

2 tablespoons coconut sugar

¼ cup canned full-fat coconut milk *or* any unsweetened plant milk

1 teaspoon vanilla extract

Small pinch of fine sea salt

Optional Flavor Boosters

¼ teaspoon espresso powder

¼ teaspoon cinnamon and/or

1–2 tablespoons melted dark chocolate for extra richness

Directions

1. Add the water, cocoa powder, maple syrup, and coconut sugar to a small saucepan and whisk until smooth.
2. Place the saucepan over medium heat and bring it to a gentle simmer, whisking to prevent lumps.
3. Add the coconut milk and continue whisking until the sauce thickens slightly, about 2 minutes.
4. Remove from heat and whisk in the vanilla and sea salt.

5. Let the sauce cool for a few minutes before using; it will thicken further as it cools.

Make It Yours Ideas

For thicker sauce, simmer an extra 2–3 minutes.

For extra rich sauce, stir in melted dark chocolate at the end.

For a deep chocolate note, add espresso powder.

To spice it up, add cinnamon or a pinch of nutmeg.

Salted Chocolate Sauce

This variation takes the base chocolate sauce and adds a deeper, rounder flavor with flaky sea salt. It's ideal for brownies, pumpkin desserts, vegan ice cream and fruit bowls.

Makes About 1 cup | Prep Time 5 minutes | Cook Time 5 minutes

Ingredients

Use the same ingredients from the regular Chocolate Sauce recipe above, with these adjustments:

- Increase the sea salt to ¼ teaspoon fine sea salt stirred in at the end
- Add a pinch of flaky sea salt on top when serving

Directions

1. Follow the same steps as the base Chocolate Sauce recipe.
2. Stir in the increased amount of sea salt after removing the sauce from heat.
3. Let it cool until it reaches your desired consistency.
4. Sprinkle flaky salt on top when serving, if desired.

Make It Yours Ideas

Use smoked flaky salt for a subtle smoky finish.

Add a splash (½ teaspoon) vanilla or caramel extract for depth.

Orange Infused Chocolate Sauce

This citrus-rich variation brightens the chocolate with fresh orange notes. It pairs beautifully with fruit trays, crepes, pancakes, and vanilla desserts.

Makes About 1 cup | Prep Time 5 minutes | Cook Time 5 minutes

Ingredients

Use the same ingredients from the regular Chocolate Sauce recipe, with these additions:

- 1 teaspoon finely grated orange zest
- 2 tablespoons fresh orange juice (replace 2 tablespoons of the water with orange juice)
- ⅛ teaspoon orange extract for stronger citrus aroma (optional)

Directions

1. Add the water, orange juice, cocoa powder, maple syrup, and coconut sugar to a small saucepan and whisk until smooth.
2. Place the saucepan over medium heat and bring to a gentle simmer.
3. Add the coconut milk and continue whisking until slightly thickened.
4. Remove from heat and stir in the vanilla, orange zest, and sea salt.
5. Let cool briefly before serving.

Make It Yours Ideas

Add a pinch of cinnamon for a warm chocolate-orange profile.

For a bolder citrus finish, double the orange zest.

Mint Chocolate Sauce

Cooling and refreshing, this variation uses peppermint extract to create a smooth chocolate-mint finish perfect for ice cream, brownies, hot cocoa toppers, and holiday desserts.

Makes About 1 cup | Prep Time 5 minutes | Cook Time 5 minutes

Ingredients

Use the same base recipe ingredients, with these additions:

- ¼–½ teaspoon peppermint extract added at the end
- A handful of finely chopped fresh mint leaves, stirred in after cooking, then strained out for a smooth sauce (optional)

Directions

1. Prepare the base Chocolate Sauce following the same steps.
2. Remove from heat and stir in the peppermint extract. Start with ¼ tsp and increase to taste.
3. Let cool slightly before serving.

Make It Yours Ideas

Add 1–2 tablespoons melted dark chocolate for a richer chocolate-mint flavor.

Stir in a pinch of ground vanilla or cinnamon for extra depth.

Mocha Chocolate Sauce

This version blends chocolate with coffee for a café-style mocha flavor. It's excellent drizzled over cakes, muffins, banana nice cream, or breakfast bowls.

Servings: Makes About 1 cup | Prep Time 5 minutes | Cook Time 5 minutes

Ingredients

Use the base recipe ingredients, with these adjustments:

- 2–3 teaspoons instant espresso powder dissolved into the water before heating .. OR .. replace ¼ cup of the water with strong brewed coffee
- Add ½ teaspoon vanilla extract for extra warmth (optional)

Directions

1. Whisk the water (or coffee), cocoa, maple syrup, coconut sugar, and espresso powder together in a saucepan.
2. Bring to a gentle simmer, whisking continuously.
3. Add coconut milk and simmer until slightly thickened.
4. Remove from heat and stir in vanilla and sea salt.
5. Cool briefly before serving.

Make It Yours Ideas

Increase espresso for a bolder mocha flavor.

Add a touch of cinnamon or cardamom for a spiced mocha effect.

Spiced Mexican Chocolate Sauce

This variation blends warming spices with a subtle heat, creating a deep chocolate flavor that works beautifully on brownies, churros-style snacks, roasted fruit, or your vegan vanilla ice cream.

Makes About 1 cup | Prep Time 5 minutes | Cook Time 5 minutes

Ingredients

Use the base Chocolate Sauce recipe with these additions:

- ½ teaspoon ground cinnamon
- ⅛–¼ teaspoon chili powder or cayenne pepper (adjust to taste)
- ¼ teaspoon espresso powder for richer depth (optional)

Directions

1. Whisk the water, cocoa powder, maple syrup, coconut sugar, cinnamon, and chili powder together in a saucepan.
2. Bring to a gentle simmer over medium heat, whisking continuously.
3. Add the coconut milk and continue cooking until slightly thickened.
4. Remove from heat and stir in vanilla and sea salt.
5. Let cool briefly before serving.

Make It Yours Ideas

Use smoked chili powder for a smoky heat.

Add a small pinch of nutmeg for warmth.

Maple Cinnamon Chocolate Sauce

This version leans into maple sweetness and warm cinnamon. It's ideal for pancakes, waffles, oat bowls, pumpkin desserts, and baked apples.

Makes About 1 cup | Prep Time 5 minutes | Cook Time 5 minutes

Ingredients

Use the base Chocolate Sauce recipe with these adjustments:

- Increase maple syrup to ⅔ cup
- Add ½ teaspoon ground cinnamon
- Optional: 1–2 teaspoons molasses for a deeper caramel undertone

Directions

1. Add the water, cocoa powder, increased maple syrup, coconut sugar, and cinnamon to a saucepan and whisk until smooth.
2. Bring to a gentle simmer over medium heat.
3. Add the coconut milk and whisk until slightly thickened.
4. Remove from heat; stir in vanilla and sea salt.
5. Cool slightly before serving.

Make It Yours Ideas

Add orange zest for a maple–cinnamon–orange twist.

Stir in a pinch of clove for a holiday flavor profile.

Coconut Almond Chocolate Sauce

Creamy, nutty, and lightly tropical, this variation pairs beautifully with fruit bowls, vegan ice cream, parfaits, baked bananas, and coconut-based desserts.

Makes About 1 cup | Prep Time 5 minutes | Cook Time 5 minutes

Ingredients

Use the base Chocolate Sauce recipe with these changes:

- Replace regular coconut milk with ¼ cup canned full-fat coconut milk
- Add 2 tablespoons almond butter (whisked in as it heats)
- ¼ teaspoon almond extract stirred in at the end (optional)

Directions

1. Add the water, cocoa powder, maple syrup, coconut sugar, and almond butter to a saucepan and whisk until combined.
2. Bring to a gentle simmer over medium heat, stirring to smooth out the almond butter.
3. Add the coconut milk and simmer until slightly thickened.
4. Remove from heat and stir in vanilla, almond extract (if using), and sea salt.
5. Let cool briefly before serving.

Make It Yours Ideas

Add shredded coconut on top when serving.

Add a tablespoon of melted dark chocolate for extra richness.

23. Herbs

Herbs are the heartbeat of flavor. They brighten, balance, and transform even the simplest vegan meals into something remarkable.

They are your kitchen's quiet teachers — teaching freshness, restraint, and creativity. This section helps you understand when to use them fresh, when to dry them, and how to make their bright flavors last.

- Fresh vs. Dried: When and Why
- Infusing Oils and Dressings with Herbs
- Growing and Storing Fresh Herbs
- Herb Pairing Guide

Fresh vs. Dried: When and Why

Fresh herbs bring vibrancy and aroma. Use them at the end of cooking or as a garnish so their delicate oils don't burn away.

Dried herbs deliver concentrated flavor and depth. Add them earlier in cooking so they have time to bloom.

A *Rule of Thumb* is to use about three times more fresh herbs than dried. For example, 1 teaspoon dried oregano ≈ 1 tablespoon fresh oregano.

Infusing Oils and Dressings with Herbs

Infused oils and dressings add a subtle herbal note that lasts beyond fresh garnishes.

Simple Infused Oil

1 cup olive oil + 1–2 sprigs of fresh herb (rosemary, thyme, or basil).
Warm gently for 5 minutes, let steep 30 minutes, then strain.
Store in a sealed bottle and use within two weeks.

Quick Herb Dressing Tip

Add fresh herbs (like parsley or cilantro) directly to your vinaigrette before shaking — it releases both flavor and color.

Growing and Storing Fresh Herbs

Grow in small pots near sunlight — most herbs (like basil, mint, parsley) thrive indoors year-round.

To store fresh tender herbs (parsley, cilantro, basil), trim stems and store in a glass of water like a bouquet; loosely cover with a plastic bag.

To store fresh hardy herbs (thyme, rosemary, sage), wrap in a slightly damp paper towel and refrigerate in a sealed bag.

To freeze the excess, blend the herbs with olive oil, freeze in ice cube trays, and use the cubes to start sauces or sautés.

Herb Pairing Guide

Use this quick reference to match herbs with their ideal companions.

Basil – Sweet, Slightly Peppery

Tomatoes, pasta sauces, tofu, balsamic, lemon

Thyme – Earthy, Floral

Mushrooms, potatoes, soups, lentils

Rosemary – Piney, Strong

Roasted vegetables, tempeh, focaccia

Oregano – Savory, Warm

Tomato sauces, Mediterranean dishes, beans

Parsley – Fresh, Clean

Grain salads, vinaigrettes, lemon-based sauces

Cilantro – Bright, Citrusy

Lime dressings, tacos, curries

Dill – Tangy, Grassy

Potatoes, vegan yogurt, lemon sauces

Mint – Cool, Sweet

Peas, fruit salads, coconut-lime dishes

Chives – Mild Onion Flavor

Dressings, tofu scrambles, dips

Sage – Warm, Woodsy

Creamy sauces, cashew blends, roasted squash

Tarragon – Slightly Anise, Sweet

Cream sauces, vinaigrettes, asparagus

24. Spices

Spices add depth, warmth, and identity to your dishes. Understanding them transforms everyday cooking into creative play.

Learn how to layer them, balance their intensity, and build your own signature blends for everything from curries to roasted vegetables.

The Role of Spices in Vegan Cooking

Spices create balance and excitement in plant-based meals.

- Warm spices (cumin, paprika, coriander) bring earthiness and body.
- Bright spices (turmeric, chili, ginger) lift flavors with color and heat.
- Sweet spices (cinnamon, cardamom) round out sauces and baked dishes.

Tip: Toast whole spices for 30–60 seconds before grinding or cooking to release their natural oils and intensifies flavor.

A Plantsy Kitchen Spice Rack

Cumin

Earthy base note for curries, soups and roasted vegetables

Smoked Paprika

Adds depth to sauces, BBQ glazes and chili

Turmeric

Brightens color and supports balance in curries and dressings

Coriander

Light and citrusy; enhances lentil or grain dishes

Ginger

Fresh or dried, it adds spice and warmth

Cinnamon

Sweet or Savory — ideal for sauces, marinades or oat bowls

Cayenne

Brings heat and sharpness; use sparingly

Black Pepper

Sharp and essential; freshly ground for the best aroma

Garlic and Onion Powder

Reliable base for sauces, dips and dressings

Italian Herb Blend

A versatile, balanced mix that complements tomato sauces, marinades, and roasted vegetables.

Makes About ½ cup

Ingredients

2 tablespoons dried oregano

1 tablespoon dried basil

1 tablespoon dried thyme

1 tablespoon dried parsley

2 teaspoons garlic powder

1 teaspoon red pepper flakes (optional)

1 teaspoon dried rosemary, crushed

Directions

Combine all ingredients and store in an airtight jar. Shake before use.

Pairs With

Marinara, roasted eggplant, or flatbread toppings.

Curry Spice Blend

Warm, golden, and fragrant — a core blend for curries, lentils, soups, or roasted vegetables.

Makes About ½ cup

Ingredients

2 tablespoons ground turmeric

1 tablespoon ground cumin

1 tablespoon ground coriander

1 tablespoon ground ginger

2 teaspoons paprika

1 teaspoon cinnamon

½ teaspoon cayenne (optional)

Directions

Whisk together and store in a sealed jar away from light.

Pairs With

Coconut Curry Cashew Sauce, lentil soups, or tofu scrambles.

Smoky BBQ Rub

Perfect for grilled or roasted vegetables, cauliflower wings, or tempeh skewers.

Makes About ½ cup

Ingredients

2 tablespoons smoked paprika

1 tablespoon chili powder

1 tablespoon brown sugar or coconut sugar

1 tablespoon garlic powder

1 teaspoon onion powder

1 teaspoon ground cumin

½ teaspoon black pepper

½ teaspoon salt

Directions

Mix well and store in a small jar. Sprinkle on before baking, grilling, or roasting.

Pairs With

BBQ sauces, baked tofu, or veggie burgers.

Sweet Spice Mix

A warm, aromatic blend that bridges breakfast and dessert — ideal for porridges, baked fruits, or energy bites.

Makes About ½ cup

Ingredients

2 tablespoons cinnamon

1 tablespoon nutmeg

1 tablespoon ground ginger

1 teaspoon cardamom

1 teaspoon allspice

½ teaspoon ground cloves

Directions

Combine all ingredients and whisk until uniform. Store tightly sealed.

Pairs With

Smoothies, oat bowls, roasted squash, or spiced hummus.

25. Nuts and Seeds

The quiet powerhouse of vegan cooking — adding creaminess, crunch, and natural richness to every dish.

The ultimate building blocks of vegan texture and flavor — nuts and seeds are your best friends in both savory and sweet dishes. Here you'll learn how to toast, grind, and transform them into butters, milks, sprinkles, and more.

Nuts and seeds bring three essential elements to vegan meals:

1. Texture – From creamy sauces to crisp toppings.
2. Flavor – Naturally buttery, toasty, and satisfying.
3. Nutrition – Protein, healthy fats, minerals, and fiber in every bite.

Use them raw for neutral flavor, roasted for depth, or blended for creaminess.

How to Toast, Grind and Store

Toast

Spread nuts or seeds in a single layer on a baking sheet. Toast at 350°F for 5–10 minutes, shaking halfway through. Watch closely — they can burn quickly. Toasting deepens flavor and enhances aroma.

Grind

Use a food processor or spice grinder for smaller batches. Pulse until desired texture — coarse for toppings, fine for butter or flour.

Store

Keep raw or toasted nuts and seeds in airtight jars in a cool, dark pantry for up to 3 months, or refrigerate for longer freshness.

Top Nuts and Seeds

Cashews – Mild, Buttery

Cream sauces, dressings, dessert

Almonds – Slightly Sweet, Crunchy

Blends, nut milks, roasted toppings

Walnuts – Earthy, Bold

Pestos, spreads, salads

Pecans – Sweet, Rich

Crumbles, desserts, roasted veggies

Sunflower Seeds – Nut Free, Toasty

Dressings, dips, granolas

Pumpkin Seeds (Pepitas) – Nutty, Dense

Toasted toppings, pestos

Sesame Seeds – Aromatic, Oily

Tahini, Asian sauces, toppings

Flaxseeds – Earthy, Mild

Smoothies, baking, egg replacer

Chia Seeds – Mild, Gelatinous

Pudding, thickening, dressings

Homemade Nut or Seed Butter

Creamy and customizable — perfect for toast, sauces, or snacks.

Makes About 2 cups

Ingredients

2 cups roasted nuts or seeds (almonds, cashews, sunflower, etc.)

Pinch of salt

1 teaspoon maple syrup (optional for sweetness)

Directions

Blend in a food processor 5–10 minutes, stopping to scrape sides as needed, until smooth and glossy. Adjust salt and sweetness to taste.

Make It Yours Ideas

Add cinnamon, cacao, or a few drops of vanilla.

Quick Nut Milk (No Soak Version)

A fresh, additive-free milk alternative — creamy and balanced.

Makes About 4 cups

Ingredients

1 cup nuts or seeds, such as cashews or almonds)

4 cups filtered water

1–2 teaspoons maple syrup (optional)

Pinch of salt

Directions

Blend all ingredients for 1–2 minutes until smooth. Strain through a nut milk bag (optional). Refrigerate for 3 days. Shake before use.

Make It Yours Ideas

Add vanilla or a pinch of cinnamon for flavor.

Savory Nut and Seed Sprinkle

A crunchy, umami-rich topping for soups, salads, and bowls.

Makes About 2 cups

Ingredients

½ cup sunflower seeds
½ cup pumpkin seeds
¼ cup sesame seeds
¼ cup poppy seeds
1 tablespoon nutritional yeast
½ teaspoon smoked paprika
½ teaspoon garlic powder
¼ teaspoon salt
¼ teaspoon crushed red pepper (optional)
¼ teaspoon cumin (optional)

Note

Adjust seeds and add nuts as desired, depending upon uses.

Directions

Toast all seeds in a dry skillet 3–5 minutes, stirring often. Stir in nutritional yeast, paprika, garlic powder, salt and crushed red pepper or cumin, if using. Cool before storing.

Uses-Sweet

Sprinkle on plant-based yogurt or oatmeal

Blend into smoothies for added protein and fiber.

Snack on them plain or in trail mix.

Uses- Savory

Sprinkle on salads, soups or plant-based pizza.

Use as a coating for tofu.

Grind flaxseeds and use to bind bean or veggie burgers.

Sweet Spice Nut Crumble

A crunchy, slightly sweet topping for oatmeal, smoothie bowls, or baked fruit.

Makes About 2 cups

Ingredients

1 cup chopped pecans or almonds

¼ cup pumpkin seeds

1 tablespoon coconut oil

2 tablespoons maple syrup

1 teaspoon cinnamon

Pinch of salt

Directions

Mix all ingredients in a bowl. Toast in a skillet over medium heat 5 minutes, stirring often, until golden and fragrant. Cool completely before storing.

Make It Yours Ideas

Add shredded coconut or cacao nibs.

26. Infused Waters

Refreshing, beautiful, and full of subtle flavor — ideal for mindful sipping or serving at the table.

Flavor doesn't always have to come from cooking — sometimes, it's as simple as what's in your glass. Infused waters add a gentle lift to hydration, with natural combinations of fruit, herbs, and citrus that refresh without sweetness.

- Cucumber-Mint-Lime Water
- Strawberry-Basil Water
- Citrus-Ginger Water
- Pineapple-Mint Water
- Blueberry-Lavendar Water

Each blend is easy to prepare, visually beautiful, and meant to be refilled throughout the day. They're a reminder that wellness lives in small choices — one sip, one moment, one infusion at a time.

Each recipe Makes About 2 quarts and can be refilled once using the same fruit and herbs. Chill for at least 2 hours before serving.

Cucumber-Mint-Lime Water

Cool, crisp, and hydrating — the classic spa water, plantsy style.

½ cucumber, thinly sliced

1 lime, thinly sliced

8–10 fresh mint leaves

Strawberry-Basil Water

Lightly sweet and aromatic with a hint of herbal freshness.

1 cup sliced strawberries

5–6 basil leaves

2 quarts filtered water

Citrus-Ginger Water

Energizing and restorative — great first thing in the morning.

1 orange, sliced

1 lemon, sliced

4 thin slices fresh ginger

Pineapple-Mint Water

Naturally sweet, tropical, and perfectly refreshing.

1 cup chopped fresh pineapple

6 mint leaves

Optional: squeeze of lime juice

Blueberry-Lavender Water

Delicate and calming — a beautiful evening sipper.

½ cup fresh blueberries (lightly crushed)

½ teaspoon dried culinary lavender (in tea infuser or sachet)

27. Bringing It All Together

Now that your staples are ready, it's time to combine them into complete, balanced, beautiful meals.

You've built your staples — now let's use them. This final section shows how to mix, match, and layer everything you've made into satisfying meals for any mood or moment. Because once you master your flavors, you'll never have to ask, *"What's for dinner?"* again.

How to Combine Sauces, Dressings and Add-Ons

Every meal begins with a base, a flavor layer, and a finish. Think of it like building a bowl from the ground up:

1. Start with the base: grains, greens, noodles, or roasted vegetables.
2. Add your protein: tofu, tempeh, beans, or lentils.
3. Layer the flavor: one sauce + one dressing or drizzle.
4. Finish with texture: toasted nuts, seeds, or a quick sprinkle.

Quick Flavor Maps

- Roasted sweet potatoes + quinoa + BBQ sauce + Lemon Herb Oil drizzle + Sunflower Seeds.
- Brown rice + chickpeas + Coconut Curry Cashew Sauce + fresh cilantro.
- Pasta + Silken Tofu Alfredo + Garlic Confit + basil and black pepper.
- Mixed greens + grilled tempeh + Tahini Drizzle + chopped walnuts.

Sample "Staples Week"

Use your sauces and staples to build a week of effortless, balanced meals.

Day 1

Lemon-Dill Cashew Sauce + roasted carrots + quinoa + chickpeas.

Day 2

Smoky Tofu Cream + BBQ cauliflower wings + brown rice.

Day 3

Mediterranean Olive and Capers Sauce + pasta + side salad with Apple Cider Maple Dressing.

Day 4

Garlic Tahini Cashew Cream + roasted broccoli + tofu + chili-lime drizzle.

Day 5

Creamy Basil Tofu Sauce + spaghetti squash + toasted walnuts.

Day 6

Coconut-Lime Drizzle + lentils + sautéed kale + lemon zest.

Day 7

Classic Marinara + grilled tempeh + Balsamic Swirl + garlic confit toast.

The "Make It Yours Ideas" Customization Guide

A reminder that your kitchen is a creative lab. Once you have your staples ready, remix them effortlessly:

- Turn Cashew Cream into Lemon-Dill Sauce by adding herbs and lemon.
- Transform Tahini Drizzle into a Spicy Harissa Sauce with chili paste.
- Blend leftover Roasted Red Pepper Sauce with beans for a quick dip.
- Add Coconut-Lime Drizzle to soup for instant brightness.
- Combine BBQ Sauce with Smoky Tofu Cream for a rich glaze.

Tip: Keep a few sauces in small jars in the fridge each week — one creamy, one spicy, one sweet, and one fresh — and mix and match as needed.

Conversion and Measurement Reference

Because clarity builds confidence:

- 1 tablespoon = 3 teaspoons
- 1 cup = 8 fluid ounces
- 1 pound = 16 ounces
- Oven conversions: 350°F ≈ 175°C, 400°F ≈ 200°C
- Storage guide:
  - Most sauces and drizzles keep 5–7 days in the fridge.
  - Oils, glazes, and spice blends can last 2–3 weeks (or longer if sealed tightly).

Closing Notes

Every sauce in this book is a building block — but what you build is entirely your own. With a few fresh herbs, toasted seeds, and a drizzle of something creamy, every meal becomes an act of creation.

Your kitchen doesn't need to be fancy — just *plantsy*, flavorful and uniquely yours.

The Clean Eats Street Playbook

If you enjoy this book and would like great plant-based meal ideas and more meal planning tools, visit Clean Eats Street. I have lots of recipes and meal planning resources available to make it easy to get organized in the kitchen. While visiting, sign up for our Farmers Market Finds newsletter to get information on what's fresh and in season each month.

Kate Witkowski

www.cleaneatsstreet.com

Thank you for Reading!

Clean Eats Street

Made in United States
North Haven, CT
06 November 2026

21793612R00157